Disordered Eating Among Athletes

A Comprehensive Guide for Health Professionals

Katherine A. Beals, PhD, RD, FACSM

Human Kinetics

Library of Congress Cataloging-in-Publication Data

Beals, Katherine A.
  Disordered eating among athletes : a comprehensive guide for health
professionals / Katherine A. Beals.
        p. ; cm.
Includes bibliographical references and index.
  ISBN 0-7360-4219-9 (hard cover)
  1. Eating disorders. 2. Athletes--Nutrition. 3. Athletes--Mental
health.
  [DNLM: 1. Eating Disorders--diagnosis. 2. Eating
Disorders--prevention & control. 3. Sports--psychology. WM 175 B366d
2004] I. Title.
  RC552.E18B43 2004
  616.85'26--dc22

                                                              2003026044

ISBN: 0-7360-4219-9

The author and publisher do not imply that the athletes appearing in the photos in this book have
eating disorders. The photos are for illustrative purposes only.

The Web addresses cited in this text were current as of February 17, 2004, unless otherwise
noted.

Acquisitions Editor: Michael S. Bahrke, PhD; **Developmental Editor:** D.K. Bihler; **Assistant
Editor:** Amanda S. Ewing; **Copyeditor:** Karen Bojda; **Proofreader:** Pam Johnson; **Indexer:** Betty
Frizzéll; **Permission Manager:** Dalene Reeder; **Graphic Designer:** Nancy Rasmus; **Graphic
Artist:** Denise Lowry; **Photo Manager:** Kareema McLendon; **Cover Designer:** Jack W. Davis;
Art Manager: Kelly Hendren; **Illustrator:** Kelly Hendren; **Printer:** Sheridan Books

Printed in the United States of America   10 9 8 7 6 5 4 3 2 1

Human Kinetics
Web site: www.HumanKinetics.com

United States: Human Kinetics, P.O. Box 5076, Champaign, IL 61825-5076
800-747-4457
e-mail: humank@hkusa.com

Canada: Human Kinetics, 475 Devonshire Road Unit 100, Windsor, ON N8Y 2L5
800-465-7301 (in Canada only)
e-mail: orders@hkcanada.com

Europe: Human Kinetics, 107 Bradford Road, Stanningley, Leeds LS28 6AT, United Kingdom
+44 (0) 113 255 5665
e-mail: hk@hkeurope.com

Australia: Human Kinetics, 57A Price Avenue, Lower Mitcham, South Australia 5062
08 8277 1555
e-mail: liaw@hkaustralia.com

New Zealand: Human Kinetics, Division of Sports Distributors NZ Ltd.,
P.O. Box 300 226 Albany, North Shore City, Auckland
0064 9 448 1207
e-mail: blairc@hknewz.com

contents

preface

Since the early 1980s there has been a growing body of literature documenting eating disturbances and body weight issues in athletes. While the plight of athletes with disordered eating has long held the interest of the scientific community, it did not gain widespread attention until Christy Henrich's much-publicized battle with, and eventual death from, anorexia nervosa. The death of this 22-year-old Olympic gymnastics hopeful seemed to open the door to the eating disorder closet as several well-recognized athletes, including Olympic gymnasts Cathy Rigby and Nadia Comaneci, Olympic swimmer Dara Torres, professional tennis player Zina Garrison, and NFL defensive end Dennis Brown, began to reveal their own personal struggles with anorexia and bulimia. Less highly publicized, yet probably much more prevalent, are the myriad athletes, both elite and recreational, suffering from partial or subclinical eating disorders. While athletes with subclinical eating disorders may not suffer the severe, life-threatening medical complications of those with clinical eating disorders, they may nevertheless experience considerable psychological distress, poor nutritional status, and compromised health.

Current estimates of the prevalence of disordered eating in athletes range from as low as 1% to as high as 62%, depending on the athletic population studied, the sport or sports examined, the definitions of disordered eating used, and the assessment techniques employed. Although there are wide variations in methodologies used, most studies have chosen to examine disordered eating in collegiate athletes. In arguably the largest U.S. survey to date, Johnson, Powers, and Dick (1999) examined the prevalence of disordered eating in 1,445 collegiate athletes (n = 883 men and n = 562 women) from 11 NCAA Division I schools. The results indicate that while only a small percentage of the athletes met the diagnostic criteria for a clinical eating disorder (1.1% of the female and none of the male athletes), a disturbingly large percentage demonstrated disordered eating behaviors (9.2%-58% of the female and .01%-38% of the male athletes).

This study and others like it leave little doubt that disordered eating among athletes is becoming increasingly common. Unfortunately, the response to this growing problem continues to lag behind its significance.

Anecdotal reports indicate that athletic administrators recognize the need to address the issue of disordered eating in athletes but are unsure of how and where to start. Athletic support staff (athletic trainers and team physicians), considered the primary authority on the topic, frequently lack the knowledge or experience necessary to properly treat athletes with disordered eating. Coaches, long accused of being both instigators and perpetuators of disordered eating in athletes, are becoming increasingly open to prevention and intervention efforts but are generally not well educated in the area of eating disorders and lack certainty about their role. Even the athletes themselves are becoming more cognizant of the potential ill effects of disordered eating on health and performance and are seeking information and guidance. Thus, now more than ever there is a need for current and accurate information on disordered eating in athletes. This book was conceived to help meet this need, to fill the informational void about athletes suffering from disordered eating.

The Purpose of This Book

The aim in writing this book was to synthesize and evaluate the current research on disordered eating in athletes, with the primary goal of bridging the gap between the scientific literature and the practical application of this information. Although this book is appropriate for anyone interested in disordered eating in athletes, it was written primarily for health, fitness, and sports professionals. More specifically, the primary audiences include the following groups (in no particular order):

- Athletic trainers or sports medicine specialists working with athletes or athletic teams or teaching future athletic trainers or sports medicine specialists

- Athletic administrators and coaches who are already familiar with the topic of disordered eating in athletes and are seeking more up-to-date, in-depth information

- Health and fitness professionals, personal trainers, and dietitians who routinely work with or counsel athletes or active individuals

- Undergraduate and graduate students enrolled in nutrition, sport psychology, exercise science, health, or wellness programs with an interest in disordered eating in athletes

How This Book Is Organized

Disordered Eating in Athletes is organized into three parts. Part I, "The Nature and Scope of Disordered Eating Among Athletes," includes chapters on disordered eating categories as they pertain to athletes, the prevalence and pathogenesis of disordered eating in athletes, and potential gender differences in disordered eating among athletes. Collectively, these chapters provide a perspective on the magnitude of the problem and show how various factors can converge to place athletes at risk for disordered eating. Part II, "Effects of Disordered Eating," addresses the wide-ranging, negative effects that disordered eating can have on the athlete. The effects of chronic energy restriction, pathogenic weight-control behaviors, and low body weight on the athlete's health and performance are discussed in detail. Specific attention is given to those ailments particularly relevant to athletes, such as loss of lean body mass and subsequent reduction in muscular strength and endurance, menstrual dysfunction, low bone mineral density, and increased susceptibility to injury. In part III, "Managing Disordered Eating in Athletes," the information in the previous chapters is integrated into a comprehensive picture of how to prevent and manage disordered eating in athletes. The focus is on education and prevention as well as treatment protocols specific to athletes and the athletic setting.

To facilitate understanding of the topics presented and to aid in using this book as an adjunct classroom text, each chapter begins with a list of objectives and concludes with a summary of pertinent points. Tables and figures are utilized throughout the chapters to synthesize and condense the information, thereby making it more manageable for the busy health professional. In addition, sidebars in some chapters provide additional information on a topic or critically evaluate a misconception or controversy surrounding disordered eating. Finally, the text concludes with a series of appendixes that provide practical information essential for individuals working with athletes who suffer from disordered eating. They include case studies, educational resources about eating disorders, nutritional guidelines, and screening surveys.

Some members of the scientific and athletic communities believe that the issue of disordered eating in athletes has been blown out of proportion, while others maintain that it is a highly significant problem currently receiving far too little attention. It is the intent of this book to bring some clarity and perhaps resolution to this important and now highly publicized issue and to address unresolved clinical and research issues in need of further study.

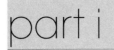

part i

Nature and Scope of Disordered Eating Among Athletes

one

Disordered Eating Categories and Their Application to Athletes

CHAPTER OBJECTIVES

After reading this chapter, you will be able to

- define and differentiate the terms *eating disorder* and *disordered eating;*

- define anorexia nervosa, bulimia nervosa, eating disorders not otherwise specified (EDNOS), and subclinical eating disorder; and

- identify the similarities and differences between athletes and nonathletes with disordered eating.

The terms *eating disorder* and *disordered eating* are frequently, yet mistakenly, used interchangeably both in the literature and in general practice. Strictly speaking, *eating disorder* refers to one of the three clinically diagnosable conditions—anorexia nervosa, bulimia nervosa, or eating disorders not otherwise specified (EDNOS)—recognized in the American Psychiatric Association's (1994) *Diagnostic and Statistical Manual of Mental Disorders* (DSM-IV). To be diagnosed with a *clinical* eating disorder, an individual must meet the criteria outlined in the DSM-IV. *Disordered eating*, on the other hand, is a general term used to describe the spectrum of abnormal and harmful eating behaviors that are used in a misguided attempt to lose weight or maintain an abnormally low or unhealthy body weight (Otis et al. 1997). Researchers and practitioners have likened the range of disordered eating behaviors as a continuum (Fries 1974; Thompson and Sherman 1993). On the extremes of this behavioral continuum are the clinical eating disorders (i.e., anorexia nervosa, bulimia nervosa, and EDNOS), while in between lie a variety of disordered eating behaviors ranging in severity from limiting food groups to significantly restricting energy intake to occasionally bingeing and purging (see figure 1.1).

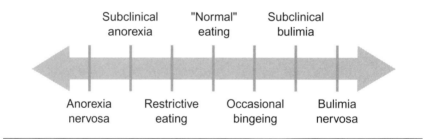

Figure 1.1   Continuum of disordered eating.

Given Americans' interest in being fit and the widespread practice of dieting, it can sometimes be difficult to tell where disordered eating stops and a clinical eating disorder begins. The following discussion attempts to clarify this distinction by describing the range of disordered eating behaviors and conditions and provides some practical tips for distinguishing these disorders in athletes.

The Clinical Eating Disorders

According to the DSM-IV (APA 1994), the clinical eating disorders—anorexia nervosa, bulimia nervosa, and EDNOS—are characterized by *severe* disturbances in eating behavior and body image. It must be emphasized that the clinical eating disorders are *psychiatric conditions*. As such, they go beyond simple body weight or shape dissatisfaction and involve more than just abnormal eating patterns and pathogenic weight control behaviors. Their behaviors are extreme, illogical, and devoid of concern for consequences. For example, when faced with the real possibility of death, one anorexic was quoted as saying, "At least I will be thin enough to fit into my coffin." Individuals suffering from clinical eating disorders often experience comorbid psychological conditions, such as obsessive-compulsive disorder, depression, or anxiety disorder (Bunnell et al. 1990; Fairburn and Brownell 2001). They often come from dysfunctional families and have a history of physical and emotional abuse (Fairburn and Brownell 2001). In addition, they often display severe feelings of insecurity and worthlessness, have trouble identifying and displaying emotions, and experience difficulty in forming close relationships with others (Fairburn and Brownell 2001).

Athletes suffering from clinical eating disorders resemble their non-athletic counterparts in many ways, but in some ways they may be quite different. These differences are largely a result of various factors that are unique to the athletic environment. The following sections describe in detail each of the clinical eating disorders and address characteristics and considerations that are specific to athletes.

Anorexia Nervosa

The term *anorexia nervosa* is derived from the Greek word *anorexia*, which literally means "lack of appetite" (Fairburn and Brownell 2001). Those familiar with the disorder will recognize that this definition is a paradoxical misnomer. Contrary to the term's implications, individuals with anorexia nervosa are *always* hungry; they are *starving*, yet they choose to deny their hunger. In fact, *denial* is a key characteristic of anorexia nervosa (and one that makes identification and subsequent treatment particularly difficult). Despite marked weight loss, significant emotional distress, and severe health problems, anorexics deny their disorder to the bitter end.

Another cardinal feature of anorexia nervosa is the desire for *control*—control of feelings, control of food, control of weight. This overwhelming need to control tangible things such as food and weight is hypothesized to be a result of the anorexic's inability to deal with the perceived chaos in his or her life (Fairburn and Brownell 2001; Garfinkel, Garner, and Goldbloom 1987; Hsu 1990).

The diagnostic criteria for anorexia nervosa as described in the DSM-IV are

- a significant loss of body weight, the maintenance of an extremely low body weight (85% of normal weight for height), or both;
- an intense fear of gaining weight or "becoming fat";
- severe body dissatisfaction and body image distortion; and
- amenorrhea (absence of three or more consecutive menstrual periods).

It should be noted that there are actually two subtypes of anorexia nervosa that have been identified: the restricting type and the binge-eating/

purging type. An individual with the restricting type of anorexia nervosa loses weight or maintains an abnormally low body weight by means of severe energy restriction and excessive exercise. An individual with the bingeing–purging type of anorexia nervosa also severely restricts energy intake and exercises excessively but occasionally binges and subsequently engages in compensatory purging behaviors such as self-induced vomiting or laxative or diuretic abuse to control weight (APA 1994).

Regardless of the subtype, the individual with anorexia nervosa is obsessed with the desire to be thin and intensely fears gaining weight. Indeed, the anorexic's life revolves around not eating and losing weight or maintaining an extremely low body weight. Anorexics wake up wondering how long they can go without eating, spend the day planning how to avoid eating, and go to sleep dreaming about the food they wish they could eat. No matter how thin anorexics become, they always feel fat and long to be thinner. Some anorexics report feeling fat in general (i.e., "fat all over"), while others realize they are thin but are still concerned that certain parts of their bodies, particularly the stomach, hips, and thighs, are too fat. It should be emphasized that this distortion of body image is not a conscious denial of the truth or simply a way for them to get attention; rather, anorexics truly believe that they are fat, and no amount of persuasion by friends, parents, siblings, or others can convince them otherwise. Moreover, the fear of becoming fat is not alleviated by weight loss. In fact, often the fear of fatness actually becomes magnified as the anorexic's body weight continues to diminish (APA 1994; Fairburn and Brownell 2001).

Individuals with anorexia nervosa tend to be high-achieving, goal-oriented, and perfectionistic. Yet, despite their accomplishments, anorexics generally suffer from extremely low self-esteem. This low self-esteem is thought to be a key factor fueling the obsession with body weight or, more specifically, with being thin. For anorexics, self-esteem (or lack thereof) becomes strongly and intimately tied to body weight, something that they are never satisfied with but are forever trying to change. Thus, weighing the body becomes a way of measuring their self-worth. Individuals with anorexia nervosa may weigh themselves several times per day (particularly after they have eaten to check for weight gain or after they have exercised to check for weight loss); they may obsessively measure or pinch various parts of their body to check for fatness and persistently check their appearance in mirrors or windows to look for areas of perceived fat (APA 1994).

For those with anorexia nervosa, the drive for thinness and the desire to control body weight become an overwhelming obsession. To achieve their elusive "ideal weight," anorexics tailor every aspect of their lives to the elusive quest for thinness, even at the expense of health. One of the first indications that a female anorexic's health is being compromised is the development of menstrual dysfunction. The menstrual dysfunction can take many forms, ranging from irregular cycles to occasionally skipping a cycle to the complete cessation of menstruation. Regardless of the exact form, menstrual dysfunction is considered an indicator of physiological dysfunction resulting from severe energy restriction and subsequent weight loss. Although all forms of menstrual dysfunction should be considered cause for concern, the diagnostic criterion listed in the DSM-IV is primary or secondary amenorrhea.

While there is no corresponding overt physiological sign in males, research does suggest that strenuous physical training combined with energy restriction may result in suppression of testicular function and subsequent depressed or absent testosterone production (and thus temporary infertility). Nonetheless, there is currently no diagnostic criterion listed in the DSM-IV pertaining to testosterone levels in males.

Athletes with anorexia nervosa, like their nonathletic counterparts, are generally perfectionistic and goal and achievement oriented, and they possess an overwhelming need for control. They diet stringently, and exercise compulsively, and as a result are extremely thin, yet they perceive themselves to be too fat. Indeed, what differentiates athletes with anorexia nervosa from nonathletes with the disorder is not so much personality or behavioral characteristics as it is the context within which the disorder manifests itself. Examples of the similarities and subtle yet significant differences between athletes and nonathletes with eating disorders are described in the following sections.

Rationale for Needing to Be Thin

Athletes with anorexia nervosa, like their nonathletic counterparts, are obsessed with the desire to be thin. However, unlike nonathletes with anorexia, who generally view thinness as the *only* goal, anorexic athletes strive for thinness as well as the improvement in performance that they *believe* will accompany it. This is particularly (although not exclusively) true for female athletes, especially those participating in sports that emphasize leanness. For whatever reason, these athletes have become convinced that thinness is equivalent to fitness and is vital for peak performance. They truly believe that they must be "thin to win." This belief is at least initially substantiated by the significant, albeit short-lived, improvement in performance that often accompanies weight loss (see chapter 5 for more on the effects of disordered eating on athletic performance). In the eyes of the anorexic athlete, achieving and maintaining an extremely low body weight is not a disorder but rather a requisite for optimal performance, and thus it becomes a significant part of how they define athletic success; it is a sign of strength and self-discipline. The inability to control body weight, on the other hand, is viewed as an unacceptable failure, a sign of weakness and lack of self-control.

The Athletic Identity Crisis

Athletes suffering from anorexia nervosa, like anorexic nonathletes, tend to possess low self-esteem. They also lack a strong sense of self-concept, but with the added complexity of having to come to terms with their athletic identity. That is, many athletes derive a large part of their self-concept from their sport. Consequently, their sense of self-worth, and subsequently their self-esteem, is closely tied to athletic performance. Indeed, many athletes, particularly those who began sport-specific training at an early age or who have been involved in sport-specific training for many years, define themselves in part, if not wholly, as athletes. Under these circumstances it is not hard to understand how a 17-year-old elite figure skater who began training at age 5 could easily lose herself in her sport. She has probably spent most of her life at the ice rink, forsaking normal childhood and adolescent activities in order to train for her sport. She probably has little concept of herself other than as a figure skater and feels that she has little else to offer. Athletic performance becomes the barometer by which she measures her worth, and the anorexic athlete sees low body weight as essential to optimal athletic performance. Thus, the athlete with anorexia nervosa views losing weight not only as a way to achieve that elusive "ideal" body weight but also as a means of *improving performance.* These potentially conflicting goals (i.e., maintaining a low body weight and achieving athletic success) can create overwhelming pressures for the anorexic athlete and generally serve to take most of the joy out of athletic participation. In addition, these unreconcilable goals render treatment significantly more complicated as a result of the difficulty in separating anorexic identify from athletic identity (see chapter 9).

Athletics as a Justification for Abnormal Eating and Exercise Patterns

Individuals with anorexia nervosa are notoriously adept at hiding and finding excuses for their extreme, often bizarre eating and exercising behaviors. For the athlete with anorexia nervosa, the sport setting provides not only an expanded repertoire of rationalizations but also an apparently valid context within which weight loss or low body weight as well as rigid and abnormal eating and exercise habits can be justified (Thompson and Sherman 1993).

Athletes with anorexia nervosa frequently blame the time constraints imposed by their sport as an excuse for not eating properly. For example, they may claim that the demands of daily life plus their intense training schedule leave little time for eating, or they may argue that eating before practice or competition will cause stomach upset and negatively affect performance. After practice they are usually "busy" (e.g., studying or working) and therefore cannot eat with the team. One collegiate cross-country runner suffering from anorexia nervosa admitted to running several miles for her cool-down after races (claiming that she needed the extra distance to "loosen up her legs") in order to burn some additional calories as well as avoid eating a postrace meal with her teammates. Those close to the athlete—teammates, parents, coaches—may unwittingly contribute to the athlete's eating disorder, as they tend to be more forgiving of the athlete's peculiar eating habits and are apt to chalk them up to the idiosyncrasies of being an athlete (Thompson and Sherman 1993).

Athletes are notorious for practicing rigid and often unconventional eating habits, making it difficult to distinguish eccentric eating from disordered eating. For example, many athletes consume monotonous diets, eating basically the same foods on a daily basis. Other athletes severely limit fat intake (one elite triathlete was known to rinse his cottage cheese, believing it would remove any last vestiges of fat!), eat the same foods before a race for good luck (one high school swimmer swore by the ergogenic effects of garlic and butter sandwiches), or avoid foods because of presumed ergolytic effects (many athletes still believe that dairy products cause excessive mucus production).

Similarly, the compulsive exercise that is characteristic of anorexia nervosa is also more readily hidden within the sport environment. Indeed, to be competitive, athletes must engage in intense, and what might be considered excessive, physical training, thus making it difficult to distinguish the committed athlete from the exercise-obsessed anorexic. Athletes with anorexia nervosa often engage in additional exercise outside their regular training under the pretext of improving performance. They exercise through injury and illness, fearing that taking time off will cause a loss of conditioning and, of greater concern, an increase in body weight. These fears also make it extremely difficult for athletes with anorexia nervosa to taper exercise prior to a competition or reduce training volume in the off-season. Eventually, the extreme exercise leads to injury or illness, yet the anorexic athlete continues to train, ignoring advice to rest from doctors, trainers, and coaches. If ultimately forced to curtail training, they likely become even more restrictive in their eating in an attempt to prevent any weight gain that may result from the decrease in training.

Athletics as Justification for Menstrual Dysfunction

Menstrual dysfunction among female athletes is alarmingly common, particularly among those who engage in sports that emphasize leanness or high training volume. It is estimated that between 3.4% and 66% of female athletes suffer from some form of menstrual dysfunction (compared with only 2%-5% of the general female population; Otis et al. 1997). Thus, the diagnostic criterion of amenorrhea poses some difficulty for diagnosing athletes with anorexia nervosa. While one should not assume that every athlete who suffers from menstrual dysfunction is also suffering from anorexia nervosa, menstrual dysfunction should never be ignored, for it is usually an early sign that health is being compromised (Otis et al. 1997). Moreover, athletes who are in fact suffering from anorexia nervosa may try to downplay their menstrual dysfunction, claiming that it is simply a result of intense training. Thus, the health professional who encounters a female athlete presenting with menstrual dysfunction is prudent to assess the athlete for eating disorders as well. (Additional information on prevention and identification of eating disorders is presented in chapters 7 and 8.) There is no diagnostic criterion similar to menstrual dysfunction (e.g., decreased sexual drive and functioning or reduced testosterone levels) for diagnosing male athletes with anorexia nervosa.

Bulimia Nervosa

The term *bulimia nervosa* is derived from the Greek word *boulimia,* which literally means "ox hunger" and is thought to symbolize the voracious and insatiable appetite that is characteristic of the disorder (Fairburn and Brownell 2001). Bulimia nervosa is a complex eating disorder characterized by repeated cycles of excessive and uncontrollable food consumption (i.e., bingeing) followed by attempts to get rid of the food (and thereby avoid weight gain) via self-induced vomiting, excessive exercise, or laxative or diuretic abuse (i.e., purging). The essential features of bulimia nervosa as described in the DSM-IV are

- episodes of binge eating (i.e., consuming a large amount of food in a short period) followed by purging (via laxatives, diuretics, enemas, or self-induced vomiting) that have occurred at least twice a week for three months,
- a sense of lack of control during the bingeing or purging episodes, and
- severe body image dissatisfaction and undue influence of body image on self-evaluation.

As with anorexia nervosa, two subtypes of bulimia nervosa have been identified: the purging type and the nonpurging type. The individual with the purging type of bulimia nervosa regularly engages in self-induced vomiting or the misuse of laxatives, diuretics, or enemas to compensate for her bingeing behaviors, whereas the individual with nonpurging bulimia nervosa uses other inappropriate compensatory behaviors such as fasting or excessive exercise (but does not regularly engage in self-induced vomiting or the misuse of laxatives, diuretics, or enemas) to compensate for episodes of overeating (APA 1994).

Individuals with bulimia nervosa strive for control yet lack the self-discipline of those with anorexia nervosa; thus, their control repeatedly breaks down. Like anorexics, individuals with bulimia are driven by a desire to lose weight and attain thinness; however, they often lack the rigid self-control of anorexics. Thus, while those with bulimia try to restrict food intake and may be quite successful at it over the short term, eventually hunger becomes overpowering, willpower breaks down, and they succumb to their hunger in vast, uncontrollable episodes of bingeing. Indeed, it is not uncommon for bulimics to consume in excess of 5,000 kcal in a single eating episode.

The binge leaves the bulimic feeling ashamed and anxious; thus, he or she will try to purge his or her body of the food (and the accompanying bad feelings and emotions) by vomiting, exercising excessively, or using laxatives or diuretics. The purge completes the cycle and brings an overwhelming sense of physiological and psychological relief to the bulimic (Fairburn and Brownell 2001). Some eating disorder experts maintain that it is the relief brought about by the purging that maintains the cycles of bingeing and purging and fosters the addictive aspect of bulimia nervosa (Fairburn and Brownell 2001; Polivy and Herman 1985). In the words of one bulimic patient, "It [the binge–purge cycle] is like a drug to me, and I love the high that it gives me. . . . I am addicted to it."

The binge–purge cycle embodies bulimics' complex and ambiguous relationship with food, a relationship that is quite distinct from that of the anorexic. For the individual with anorexia nervosa, food is foe, something to be feared and avoided at all costs. The individual with bulimia nervosa maintains more of a love–hate relationship with food. On one hand, food

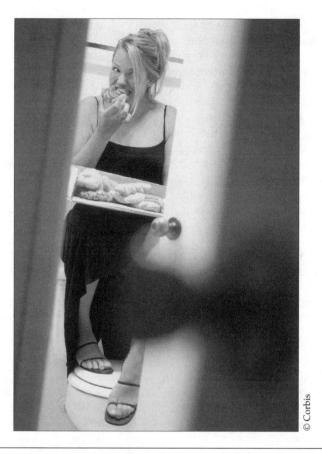

Bulimics may be successful at restricting food intake in the short term, but eventually the hunger becomes overpowering, willpower breaks down, and they succumb to their hunger in episodes of bingeing.

provides the bulimic with the comfort, pleasure, and security that is lacking in his or her life; thus, food is friend. On the other hand, food is associated with weight gain, and thus, food is also foe. One bulimic described his relationship with food this way, "When things are out of control in my life, food is there for me. When I binge, the pain, hurting, and sadness go away. But after the binge the guilt comes, and I have to get rid of it." Key to the diagnostic criteria for bulimia nervosa is the frequency with which the binge–purge cycles occur. That is, to be clinically diagnosed with bulimia nervosa, an individual must engage in binge–purge cycles at least twice a week for at least three months.

The outward appearance of the bulimic also differs markedly from that of the anorexic. For example, in sharp contrast to the emaciated appearance of anorexics, individuals with bulimia nervosa are typically of normal weight or may be slightly overweight. In addition, unlike anorexics, who are generally introverted and tend to isolate themselves from others, those with bulimia nervosa are more extroverted and outgoing. Nonetheless, while individuals with bulimia may appear self-assured and well-adjusted, they secretly harbor feelings of worthlessness and low self-esteem similar to those with anorexia. In fact, the bulimic's disorder is often so well hidden that even those closest to him or her (such as family, friends, or spouse) may fail to recognize the illness. While bulimics may keep their disordered eating behaviors well hidden, they are not particularly adept at concealing their dissatisfaction with their body weight or shape. Indeed, individuals with bulimia nervosa tend to be overly critical of their body weight or shape and are not shy about voicing their self-dissatisfaction.

Athletes with bulimia nervosa are similar to their nonathletic counterparts in many respects. Their moods, emotions, self-esteem, and body weight tend to be as erratic as their eating patterns, which, like those of bulimic nonathletes, are characterized by repeated cycles of bingeing and purging. Similarly, they are overconcerned and dissatisfied with body weight, shape, and size. Nonetheless, just as there were subtle differences between the athlete and the nonathletic individual with anorexia nervosa, so too are there slight differences between athletes and nonathletes with bulimia nervosa.

Definition of Binge and Purge

Athletes suffering from bulimia nervosa, like bulimic nonathletes, engage in regular binge–purge cycles; however, both the binge and purge may be somewhat less clearly defined when it comes to athletes. According to the DSM-IV, a binge is defined as eating "a large amount of food in a discrete period of time." As might be expected, problems arise in interpreting the phrases "large amount of food" and "discrete period of time," particularly as they apply to athletes. According to the DSM-IV, a "large amount" is defined as "larger than most individuals would eat under similar circumstances." It could be argued that, because of increased energy expenditure and therefore increased energy requirements, athletes generally consume more food than "most individuals." Moreover, the varied energy needs of athletes make it difficult to characterize or compare "similar circumstances." The context of eating must also be taken into consideration. For example, what may be thought of as excessive consumption at a typical meal might be considered normal under certain circumstances, such as carbohydrate loading for a competitive event or refueling after a particularly prolonged or intense training session.

Further complicating the issue is the objective versus subjective experience of "a large amount." No one would dispute that eating 5,000 kcal at a single sitting is a large or excessive amount. But what if the athlete eats only 500 kcal yet feels out of control while eating and extremely guilty after eating? Is this still a binge? In the objective sense (i.e., based simply on the amount of food eaten), this would not be considered a binge. However, from a subjective standpoint (i.e., the athlete's feeling out of control and the accompanying guilt), it would certainly count as a binge episode. For this reason, many eating disorder specialists maintain that the actual amount of food is not as important as the athlete's *perception* of the amount of food, particularly when it comes to eliciting the subsequent guilt and triggering the compensatory purging behaviors (APA 1994; , Fairburn and Brownell 2001). As long as an athlete believes that he or she has consumed too much food, it is a binge in his or her mind, no matter how many calories were actually consumed.

Equally confusing when interpreting the definition of a binge is the issue of time. According to the DSM-IV, a "discrete period of time" is a "limited period, usually less than 2 hours," yet once again, the DSM-IV leaves room for interpretation by further stating that a binge need not be restricted to one setting. Thus, an athlete could conceivably begin a binge in one location (e.g., the dormitory cafeteria, a restaurant, or a party) and then continue it later at another location (e.g., upon returning home) even though more than two hours have elapsed. The two-hour time period introduces another complication in interpreting a binge for the athlete. Athletes (particularly endurance athletes) are often encouraged to consume large amounts of carbohydrate-rich foods within two hours after an exercise bout in order to maximize glycogen resynthesis. This makes it difficult to determine what is a binge versus a recommended dietary practice.

Factors Precipitating the Binge–Purge Cycle

The factors precipitating binge–purge cycles and the rationalizations accompanying them also serve to differentiate athletes with bulimia nervosa from their nonathletic counterparts. Although the bulimic athlete, like the bulimic nonathlete, often restricts food intake severely during the day and engages in binge–purge behaviors later in the evening (when no one else is around), the reasons for food restriction and subsequent bingeing and purging may be somewhat distinct. For example, the bulimic nonathlete generally restricts food intake for weight loss alone, whereas food restriction for the bulimic athlete serves a dual purpose: weight loss and performance enhancement (or at least the bulimic athlete uses the guise of performance to justify food restriction). For example, she may not eat anything before a workout or competition, fearing that it will make her feel heavy and slow and negatively affect her performance. Similarly, she may not eat after practice or competition, particularly if eating with teammates, for fear that her eating will get "out of control" and that she will binge in front of her teammates and then need to find a way to secretly purge. Thus, the bulimic athlete may go all day with little or no food. By nighttime she is likely to be extremely hungry and tired, her resistance is down, and even if she does not intend to do so, she may find it very difficult to control her eating, thus precipitating a binge and subsequent purge.

Although typically triggered by periods of food restriction or dieting, the bingeing and purging cycles of the athlete with bulimia nervosa may be caused by other factors unique to the sport setting, including athletic identity, performance dynamics, and environmental cues. As is true for anorexic athletes, bulimic athletes tend to tie self-esteem and self-worth to athletic performance. Anything that threatens their athletic identity also threatens their fragile sense of self-esteem. Such threats can be very stressful, eliciting the bulimic athlete's number-one coping mechanism, bingeing and purging.

The dynamics of performance and its effect on an athlete's self-esteem can also trigger a binge–purge cycle. For example, a good performance can boost an athlete's sense of self-worth (however fleetingly), and the athlete may reward himself or herself with food, particularly forbidden foods, which may precipitate a binge and subsequent purge. A poor performance, on the other hand, is a direct blow to the athlete's fragile self-esteem, and he or she may turn to food for comfort or to help ease the agony of defeat, which ultimately leads to a binge and subsequent purge. Alternatively, an athlete may seek refuge in bingeing and purging behaviors to cope with the stress of performance, parental pressure, or difficulties with a coach or teammates (Thompson and Sherman 1993).

Finally, the athletic environment provides opportunities for bingeing that are generally not available to the nonathlete with bulimia. One of these is carbohydrate loading, a common practice among endurance athletes, which involves consuming large amounts of carbohydrate-rich foods one or two days before an endurance event. In this situation the bulimic athlete is encouraged to engage in the very behavior he or she is ashamed of and trying to avoid! Although carbohydrate loading is particularly common before a competition, it is also frequently practiced at postcompetition meals. To complicate matters further, many athletes routinely consume meals together as a team, and studies have shown that people generally consume more food when eating with peers in social settings (Anderson 1996). These environmental cues, individually or collectively, can increase the likelihood of a binge and a subsequent purge.

Fear of Being Discovered

Athletes with bulimia nervosa, like bulimic nonathletes, live in fear of being found out, and they thus tend to avoid "high-risk" situations. One particular risky situation is eating with the team. Although bulimic athletes would just as soon avoid eating with the team, to do so would certainly arouse suspicion. On the other hand, they fear that their eating will get out of control or that teammates will become suspicious of their ability to remain relatively thin despite consuming such large quantities of food. Thus, eating with the team presents a stressful dilemma for the bulimic athlete. As previously mentioned, the stress of team meals can be further compounded by the practice of carbohydrate loading. Then there is the problem of concealing the purging behaviors that inevitably follow the binge. Thus, athletes with bulimia nervosa worry about keeping eating under control, they fear that eating will get out of control, and they dread being discovered in a purge and confronted about the disorder. Road trips perhaps pose the greatest challenge for the bulimic athlete, as eating with the team is inescapable. Road trips and team meals can be stressful and can create enormous anxiety for bulimic athletes, which they are apt to try to manage through their only available coping mechanism, bingeing and purging. In fact, it has been reported that athletes with bulimia nervosa confess that they worry more about being discovered on road trips than about the competition or their performance (Thompson and Sherman 1993).

Exercise as the Predominant Purging Method

It has been suggested that athletes with bulimia nervosa are more likely to engage in excessive exercise after a binge than their nonathletic counterparts, who are more apt to purge using vomiting or laxatives (Thompson and Sherman 1993). This difference in purging behaviors is again largely

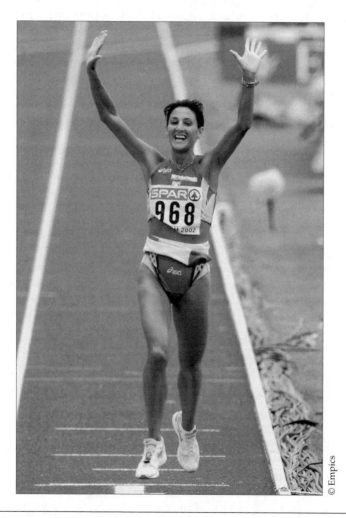

For athletes with anorexia or bulimia nervosa, losing weight is viewed not only as a way to achieve that elusive "ideal" body weight but also as a means of improving performance.

explained by the nature of the sport setting. That is, because exercise is a behavior that athletes already engage in, it is easier for bulimic athletes, like anorexic athletes, to disguise excessive physical activity or at least to rationalize it in the name of improved performance. Conversely, concealing vomiting or the use of laxatives and diuretics is much more difficult for the athlete, particularly during road trips or other team functions (Thompson and Sherman 1993).

Menstrual Dysfunction

Although not a diagnostic criterion for bulimia nervosa, menstrual dysfunction is fairly common among bulimic athletes and is thought to result from the energy drain and physiological stress elicited by the binge–purge cycles (Thompson and Sherman 1993). As is true of the anorexic athlete, the bulimic athlete often uses the intense training associated with her sport to explain away menstrual dysfunction. Thus, as recommended previously, health professionals should further assess athletes with menstrual dysfunction for the presence of an eating disorder.

Eating Disorders Not Otherwise Specified (EDNOS)

Eating disorders not otherwise specified (EDNOS) is a clinical eating disorder category that was recently added to the DSM-IV to describe conditions that meet some but not all of the criteria for anorexia nervosa and bulimia nervosa. For example, an athlete may meet all the criteria for anorexia nervosa except that his or her weight for height is normal or acceptable, despite severe energy restriction. Or the individual may meet all the criteria for bulimia nervosa except that bingeing and purging episodes occur less frequently than two times per week or have been occurring over a period of less than three months (the minimum required for a diagnosis of bulimia nervosa). EDNOS addresses these special exceptions to the better-recognized clinical conditions anorexia nervosa and bulimia nervosa. These are the characteristic features of EDNOS as described in the DSM-IV:

- All the criteria for anorexia nervosa are met except amenorrhea.
- All the criteria for anorexia nervosa are met except that, despite significant weight loss, the individual's current weight is within the normal range.
- All the criteria for bulimia nervosa are met except that the binge and purge cycles occur at a frequency of less than twice a week for a duration of less than three months.
- An individual of normal body weight regularly uses purging behaviors after eating small amounts of food (e.g., self-induced vomiting after consuming only two cookies).
- An individual repeatedly chews and spits out, but does not swallow, large amounts of food.

Disordered Eating Syndromes

In some cases athletes may exhibit all of the overt behaviors of a clinical eating disorder but do not harbor the severe psychological disturbances that underlie the disorders (Beals and Manore 1994, 1999, 2000; Smith 1980; Thompson and Sherman 1993). These partial eating disorder syndromes have been classified and characterized in a variety of ways by a number of researchers and practitioners. The most common of these classifications are outlined in the following sections.

Subclinical Eating Disorders

In one of the first studies to systematically examine the full spectrum of disordered eating behaviors, Button and Whitehouse (1981) described a population of female nonathlete college students who manifested symptoms similar to anorexia nervosa but with less severity and frequency. The authors referred to this subclinical variant of anorexia nervosa as *subclinical anorexia*. Using case study data, Smith (1980) adapted the concept of subclinical anorexia to describe a young male athlete who displayed significant body weight dissatisfaction and engaged in extreme weight loss methods in an effort to improve his performance. Eventually, the strict dieting and maintenance of an extremely low body weight were no longer the means to the end of athletic performance but became the end itself.

The term *subclinical eating disorder* has since been frequently used by researchers to describe considerable eating pathology and body weight concerns in both athletes and nonathletes who do not demonstrate significant psychopathology or who fail to meet all the DSM-IV criteria for anorexia nervosa, bulimia nervosa, or EDNOS (Beals and Manore 1994, 1999, 2000; Bunnell et al. 1990; Smith 1980; Thompson and Sherman 1993; Williamson et al. 1995; Wilmore 1991). Indeed, many athletes do not meet the technical criteria for a clinical eating disorder, despite severely restricting energy intake, engaging in self-induced vomiting, or using laxatives, diuretics, and excessive exercise in an effort to lose weight. Conversely, athletes may use none of these methods but still suffer from an obvious eating disturbance.

For example, one elite male distance runner reported routinely eating less than 2,600 kcal/d while averaging 100 miles (161 km) per week and working out at the gym almost on a daily basis. He ate similar foods every day and severely limited his fat intake (≤ 20 g/d) because he felt that he was too fat (his weight was actually on the low end of normal). Occasionally he would binge (eat too much of a forbidden food, such as a piece of cake or an order of french fries), generally when he went out to dinner with the team or after a day of severely restricting his food intake. Afterward, he would feel horribly guilty and would generally exercise twice as much the next day in order to burn off the calories (once he even went out for a run late at night to burn off a particularly large team meal). Yet he never vomited (although he thought about it once or twice) or used diuretics or laxatives. While he was openly dissatisfied with his body weight and shape, he did not display any significant emotional distress or psychological disturbance. This athlete is definitely displaying disordered eating behaviors; however, he does not meet the diagnostic criteria for anorexia nervosa or bulimia nervosa. In fact, depending on the context of the evaluation, he might not even meet the criteria necessary for a diagnosis of EDNOS.

Whether or not an athlete meets all the diagnostic criteria for one of the clinical eating disorders should not be the issue. Rather, the concern should be the extent to which the disorder is compromising the athlete's physical and mental health. The weight control behaviors of the athlete just described will no doubt eventually affect his performance and his health. Thus, despite the lack of clinical evidence, intervention and treatment are clearly warranted (more details on treatment are covered in chapter 9).

Anorexia Athletica

A prominent researcher in the area of eating disorders in athletes, Jorunn Sundgot-Borgen (1993b), has developed a set of criteria to describe a variant of anorexia nervosa in athletes that she refers to as *anorexia athletica*. Accord-

---

Essential Features of Anorexia Athletica
- Weight loss > 5% of expected body weight +
- Delayed menarche (i.e., no menstrual bleeding by age 16) (+)
- Menstrual dysfunction (amenorrhea or oligomenorrhea) (+)
- Gastrointestinal complaints (+)
- Absence of medical illness or affective disorder to explain the weight loss +
- Body image distortion (+)
- Excessive fear of weight gain or becoming obese +
- Restriction of energy intake (<1,200 kcal/d) +
- Use of purging methods (e.g., self-induced vomiting, laxatives, diuretics) (+)
- Binge eating (+)
- Compulsive exercise (+)

Criteria for Fear of Obesity
- Weight loss > 5% of expected body weight (+)
- Delayed puberty (+)
- Absence of medical illness or affective disorder to explain the weight loss
- Excessive fear of becoming obese +
- Restriction of food intake (<1,200 kcal/d) +

Figure 1.2   Features of anorexia athletica.

The criteria marked with + are considered absolute criteria, meaning that they are required for diagnosis, while the criteria marked with (+) are relative criteria and need not be present to make a diagnosis of anorexia athletica. The criteria for anorexia athletica were derived largely from a set criteria used to describe a disorder referred to as *fear of obesity* observed in a small sample of nonathletic adolescents (Pugliese et al. 1983).

ing to Sundgot-Borgen, the athlete with anorexia athletica demonstrates an intense fear of gaining weight or becoming fat even though underweight (at least 5% below the expected normal weight for age and height). This weight loss is achieved by severe energy restriction (<1,200 kcal/d), excessive exercise, self-induced vomiting, or the abuse of laxatives and diuretics (Sundgot-Borgen 1993b). The essential features of anorexia athletica are outlined in figure 1.2.

Summary

Disordered eating is a broad term encompassing a wide range of abnormal and unhealthy eating behaviors that are used in an attempt to lose weight or maintain an extremely low body weight. On the spectrum of disordered eating behaviors, the clinical eating disorders (i.e., anorexia nervosa, bulimia nervosa, EDNOS) are situated at either end, and the subclinical variants lie more toward the middle. This characterization of disordered eating behaviors implies that they are not readily distinguished from one another. Indeed, individuals suffering from disordered eating often move along the continuum, exhibiting different degrees of disordered eating and body image distortion or dissatisfaction at different points in time.

Athletes with eating disorders generally are more similar to their nonathletic counterparts than different. In fact, the subtle differences between athletes and nonathletes with eating disorders lie not in any distinct personality or behavioral characteristics but rather in the context within which the disorder manifests itself. That is, the sport setting often affords the athlete greater opportunities to justify, legitimize, and disguise the disorder. This can make identification and subsequent intervention and treatment much more difficult.

two

Prevalence of Disordered Eating Among Athletes

CHAPTER OBJECTIVES

After reading this chapter, you will be able to

■ identify the prevalence of disordered eating among athletes,

■ describe the reasons for the variability in current prevalence estimates and why they likely represent an underestimation of the actual prevalence of disordered eating among athletes, and

■ explain why disordered eating is hypothesized to be more prevalent among athletes (particularly those in thin-build sports) than nonathletes.

An Eating Disorder Epidemic?

There are likely very few health professionals who have not been exposed to disordered eating in some way, shape, or form. Professional journals, newspapers, magazines, television news shows, and daytime talk shows seem to be abuzz with the topic of disordered eating. Media coverage is particularly fierce when a celebrity, whether it be an actor or a sports figure, makes the news by admitting to having an eating disorder. In fact, the increasing interest in and publicity surrounding eating disorders might give the impression that we are in the midst of an eating disorder epidemic.

There is little doubt that as a population we are extremely dissatisfied with our bodies and are overly concerned with dieting and weight loss. It has been reported that 80% of American women are dissatisfied with their appearance and 45% are dieting to control their weight (Smolak, Levine, and Streigel-Moore 1996). Moreover, it is estimated that 35% of these so-called normal dieters may eventually develop disordered eating behaviors, and of those, 20% to 25% will progress to subclinical or even clinical eating disorders (Smolak, Levine, and Streigel-Moore 1996).

Nonetheless, despite the media hype and weight consciousness of the American public, existing data do not support the notion of an eating disorder epidemic. In fact, prevalence estimates from the most recent epidemiological studies using strict DSM-IV diagnostic criteria indicate that only 0.5% to 1.0% of young women suffer from anorexia nervosa, while approximately 1% to 3% suffer from bulimia nervosa (APA 1994; Hoek 1993). The prevalence of eating disorders not otherwise specified (EDNOS) is thought to be somewhat higher, affecting between 3% and 5% of young women (APA 1994; Byrne and McLean 2001). Although exact prevalence estimates of eating disorders in men are not currently available, the limited data available suggest a rate of occurrence that is approximately 1/10 of that in women (Hoek 1993, 1995; Shisslak, Crago, and Estes 1995).

It should be noted that the shame and secrecy surrounding eating disorders likely cause many cases to go unreported. Thus, the prevalence estimates presented in the preceding paragraph likely underestimate the true prevalence of eating disorders among women and men in the United States. Moreover, these prevalence estimates do not include the potentially significant number of individuals with partial or subclinical eating disorders or who engage in disordered eating behaviors. Thus, the true prevalence of disordered eating among the U.S. population is likely much higher than current estimates suggest.

Disordered Eating Prevalence Among Athletes: Why So Many Numbers?

Current estimates of the prevalence of disordered eating among athletes are highly variable, ranging from less than 1% to as high as 62% in female athletes (Brownell and Rodin 1992; Byrne and McLean 2001; Otis et al. 1997) and between 0% and 57% in male athletes (Andersen 1992; Byrne and McLean 2001). A summary of the studies that have examined the prevalence of disordered eating among female and male athletes is presented in table 2.1.

There are at least three reasons for the large variation in eating disorder prevalence estimates among athletes: (1) sample characteristics, (2) definition of eating disorder used, and (3) methods of assessing eating disorders.

Sample Characteristics

Most studies investigating the prevalence of disordered eating among athletes are limited by very small and restricted samples (i.e., a small number of athletes representing one or maybe two sports). Indeed, only four of the studies presented in table 2.1 used a sufficiently large sample of athletes (>200) representing multiple sports (Beals and Manore 2002; Black and Burkes-Miller 1988; Johnson, Powers, and Dick 1999; Sundgot-Borgen 1993b). The remainder either employed inadequate sample sizes or examined single sports, both of which can bias prevalence estimates. For example, prevalence estimates derived from an investigation of a "thin-build" sport, or one that is known to be at high risk for disordered eating (e.g., ballet, gymnastics, cross-country running), are likely to be higher than those from sports considered to impart lesser risk (e.g., basketball, field hockey, soccer).

Studies have also been somewhat inconsistent in the subjects they have recruited and labeled *athletes*. Table 2.1 clearly shows that the term *athlete* has been used to describe a wide range of individuals of varying levels of athletic ability and sport participation. For example, some studies used collegiate athletes, others used elite (Olympic-caliber) athletes, and still others used high school, recreational, or club athletes. In fact, some studies did not even specify the type of athlete used! These inconsistencies in sample characteristics surely produce varying estimates of disordered eating prevalence.

Definition of Eating Disorder

Studies examining the prevalence of eating disorders among athletes have varied widely in their definitions of the term *eating disorder*. While some studies adhered to the strict DSM-IV diagnostic criteria, most used the clinical term *eating disorder* to characterize a wide range of abnormal eating behaviors that would be more appropriately labeled *disordered eating*. Of course, using stricter diagnostic criteria (such as those outlined in the DSM-IV) will produce a lower prevalence estimate than using more liberal classification criteria. For example, using the DSM-III diagnostic criteria, Sundgot-Borgen (1993b) found that 1.3% and 8.0% of female athletes suffered from anorexia nervosa and bulimia nervosa, respectively. In contrast, using pathogenic weight control methods as the diagnostic criteria , Rosen et al. (1986) reported a significantly higher "eating disorder" prevalence rate among female collegiate athletes of 32%.

Table 2.1 Summary of Studies on Prevalence of Disordered Eating in Athletes

Study	Subjects	Instrument	Findings
Multiple sports			
Beals and Manore (2002)	425 female collegiate athletes	EAT-26 and EDI-BD	3.3% and 2.4% of the athletes self-reported a diagnosis of clinical anorexia and bulimia nervosa, respectively; 15% and 31.5% of the athletes scored above the designated cutoff scores on the EAT-26 and EDI-BD, respectively (indicative of disordered eating).
Black and Burkes-Miller (1988)	695 collegiate athletes (382 men from 8 different sports and 313 women from 7 different sports)	Questionnaire developed by the authors to determine prevalence of pathogenic weight control behaviors	21.4% of men and 25.1% of women ate <600 kcal/d; 6.6% and 14.7% respectively used fasting; 7.3% and 13.4% respectively used fad diets; 3.5% and 7.3% respectively used self-induced vomiting; 2.9% and 4.5% respectively used laxatives; 1.9% and 4.2% respectively used diuretics; 1.9% and 1.0% respectively used enemas.
Davis and Cowles (1989)	126 female athletes, 64 in thin-build (TB) sports, 62 in normal-build (NB) sports	EDI	89% of the athletes in TB sports and 58% in NB sports reported a desire to lose weight; 38% of the athletes in TB sports and 27% of the athletes in NB sports reported constantly dieting.
Johnson, Powers, and Dick (1999)	1445 collegiate athletes (883 men and 562 women) from 11 NCAA Division I Schools	EDI-2 and questionnaire developed by the authors using DSM-IV criteria	None of the men or women met the criteria for anorexia nervosa; none of the men and 1.1% of the women met the criteria for bulimia nervosa. 9.2% of the women and 0.01% of the men met the criteria for subclinical bulimia; 2.8% of women met the criteria for subclinical anorexia. 5.5% of the women and 2% of the men reported purging (vomiting, using laxatives or diuretics) on a weekly basis.

Study	Sample	Measure	Findings
Kurtzman et al. (1989)	126 female athletes from unspecified sports	EDI and questionnaire developed by the authors assessing eating disorder attitudes and behaviors compatible with DSM-III criteria	0.8% reported a current diagnosis of anorexia and bulimia nervosa. Several athletes reported practicing pathogenic weight control behaviors, including self-induced vomiting (9.3%), excessive and deliberate weight loss (12.7%), using laxatives (8.8%), and using diuretics (12.7%).
Rosen et al. (1986)	182 female collegiate athletes representing 10 different sports	Questionnaire developed by the authors assessing dieting practices and pathogenic weight control behaviors	32% practiced at least one pathogenic weight control behavior. The athletes were more apt to resort to pathogenic weight control behaviors if they perceived themselves to be overweight. Gymnasts and runners had the highest percentage of weight control behaviors (74% and 47% respectively).
Stoutjesdyk and Jevne (1993)	191 Canadian collegiate or "club" athletes (104 women and 87 men) representing 6 different sports	EAT-40	10.6% of women and 4.6% of men scored above the EAT cutoff. Athletes in sports that emphasize leanness scored higher on the EAT than those in sports in which a lower body weight is not considered advantageous.
Sundgot-Borgen (1993b)	522 Norwegian elite female athletes	EDI and in-depth interview developed by the author based on DSM III criteria	1.3%, 8.0%, and 8.2% were diagnosed with anorexia nervosa, bulimia nervosa, and anorexia athletica, respectively.
Sundgot-Borgen and Corbin (1987)	35 female athletes in sports emphasizing leanness and 32 in sports not emphasizing leanness	EDI	10% of all athletes and 20% of athletes in sports emphasizing leanness were highly preoccupied with weight and body image or had tendencies toward eating disorders as indicated by elevated scores on the EDI.

(continued)

Table 2.1 *(continued)*

Study	Subjects	Instrument	Findings
Sundgot-Borgen et al. (1999)	The total population of Norwegian elite athletes (960 men and 660 women) representing 60 different sporting events.	A questionnaire developed by the authors, including subscales of the EDI, weight history, and self-reported history of eating disorders	20% (*n* = 156) of the female athletes and 8% (*n* = 27) of the male athletes met the DSM-IV criteria for clinical eating disorders (i.e., anorexia nervosa, bulimia nervosa, or EDNOS).
Cheerleading			
Gottlieb et al. (1994)	621 junior and senior high school girls at the National Cheerleading Association competition	Questionnaire developed by the authors measuring factors related to eating disorders	30% and 51% of the cheerleaders reported spending a lot of time thinking about food and their weight, respectively. 6% reported a history of purging after eating. 23% reported 2 or more of these behaviors.
Lundholm and Littrell (1986)	751 female high school cheerleaders (13-18 yr) attending a 5-day cheerleading camp	Questionnaire developed by the authors (Desire for Thinness Scale), Restrained Eating Scale, EDI-BD, and EDI-Bul, and EAT-40	Those who scored in the upper third (*n* = 250) of the total population on the Desire for Thinness Scale had significantly higher scores on all but one of the eating disorder scales compared with those who scored in the lower third.
Dance			
Brooks-Gunn, Warren, and Hamilton (1987)	55 adult female ballet dancers in U.S. and European regional and national companies	EAT-26 and self-reported history of anorexia or bulimia nervosa	17% reported a history of anorexia nervosa and 21% reported a history of bulimia nervosa. Those with a history of eating disorders had higher EAT scores.

Evers (1989)	21 female university students in intermediate or advanced dance classes	EAT-40	33% had elevated EAT scores indicative of being at risk for an eating disorder.
Hamilton, Brooks-Gunn, and Warren (1985)	55 white and 11 black female dancers in national and regional companies	EAT-40 and self-reported history of anorexia or bulimia nervosa	15% and 19% of white dancers reported past or present anorexia nervosa and bulimia nervosa, respectively. None of the black dancers reported an eating disorder.
Hamilton et al. (1988)	49 female ballet dancers: 19 from highly select and 13 from less select American companies, 17 from highly select Chinese companies	EAT-26 and self-reported history of anorexia and bulimia nervosa	10% of the highly select and 46% of the less select dancers from American companies and 24% of the highly select Chinese dancers reported past or present anorexia or bulimia nervosa.
Le Grange, Tibbs, and Noakes (1994)	49 female students (16-29 yr) at a university ballet school	EAT-26, demographic and dieting history. Those scoring $\geq$ 30 on the EAT-26 underwent a clinical interview based on the DSM-III criteria.	27% had EAT-26 scores $\geq$ 30; 2 of these were diagnosed with clinical and 4 with subclinical anorexia nervosa.
Szmukler et al. (1985)	100 female ballet students (13-20 yr) at a prestigious English ballet school	EAT-26. Those scoring $\geq$ 30 underwent a physical exam and psychological interview (based on the DSM criteria).	16% scored $\geq$ 30 on the EAT-26; 7 of these were identified by physical and psychological interviews as possible cases of anorexia nervosa.

(continued)

Table 2.1 *(continued)*

Study	Subjects	Instrument	Findings
Figure skating			
Rucinski (1989)	17 male and 23 female figure skaters	EAT-40	48% of the female skaters had elevated EAT scores indicative of disordered eating. None of the male skaters had high EAT scores.
Zeigler et al. (1998)	21 young competitive female figure skaters	EAT-40	2 scored above the EAT cutoff indicating disordered eating.
Gymnastics			
O'Connor, Lewis, and Kirchner (1995)	23 female collegiate gymnasts	EDI-2 and Eating Disorder Symptom Checklist	22% had elevated EDI-2 drive for thinness scores and more than half reported using at least one pathogenic weight control method.
Petrie (1993); Petrie and Stoever (1993)	213 female collegiate gymnasts	BULIT-R	61.3% were identified as having intermediate-level disordered eating. 4.1% had BULIT-R scores indicative of bulimia. 32.6% reported binge eating at least once per week, 6% reported vomiting at least 2 times per month, and 2.4% reported using laxatives at least once per week.
Rosen and Hough (1988)	42 collegiate gymnasts	Michigan State University Weight Control Survey	62% reported using at least one pathogenic weight control method including self-induced vomiting (25%), fasting (24%), using diuretics (12%), using diet pills (24%), and using laxatives (7%).

Sundgot-Borgen (1996)	12 female rhythmic gymnasts	EDI, dietary and nutritional history	Half suffered from disordered eating: 2 met the DSM-III criteria for anorexia nervosa, 2 met the criteria for anorexia athletica, and 2 reported regularly vomiting, fasting, or using laxatives.

Rowing

Sykora et al. (1993)	162 heavyweight rowers (73 women and 89 men)	EAT-26 and self-developed questionnaire on eating, dieting, and weight control practices	20% of women and 12.3% of men reported binge eating 2 or more times per week, 57% of men and 25% of women reported fasting, and 2.5% of men and 13.2% of women reported vomiting for weight loss.
Terry, Lane, and Warren (1999)	103 elite lightweight and heavyweight rowers (44 women and 59 men)	EAT-26 and BSQ	12% of the lightweight rowers and 1 heavyweight scored above the EAT-26 cutoff. EAT-26 scores were significantly higher among lightweight than heavyweight rowers. BSQ scores were higher for heavyweights and women than for lightweights and men.

Running

Clark, Nelson, and Evans (1988)	93 elite female distance runners	Self-developed questionnaire	13% reported a history of anorexia nervosa, 25% reported undesired binge eating, and 9% stated that they binged and purged. A total of 34% reported atypical eating behaviors.
Gadpille, Sanborn, and Wagner (1987)	13 amenorrheic and 19 normally menstruating runners	Interview by a psychiatrist to establish DSM-III criteria	62% of the amenorrheic runners and none of the normally menstruating runners reported eating disorders.

(continued)

Table 2.1　(continued)

Study	Subjects	Instrument	Findings
Hulley and Hill (2001)	181 elite U.K. female distance runners	EDE-Q	29 runners (16%) reported a present diagnosis of an eating disorder (7 with anorexia nervosa, 2 with bulimia nervosa, and 20 with EDNOS). 6 runners (3%) had received previous treatment for an eating disorder.
Pasman and Thompson (1988)	90 male and female runners, weightlifters and sedentary controls	Body size estimation and 3 subscales of the EDI (EDI-BD, EDI-BUL, and EDI-DT)	Females in all groups had greater body dissatisfaction than males. Runners and weightlifters had greater eating disturbances than controls. Female runners exhibited significantly more eating psychopathology than male runners.
Weight and Noakes (1987)	125 female distance runners (85 recreational marathoners, 15 elite ultramarathoners, and 25 collegiate cross-country runners)	EAT-26 and EDI	Only 1 runner reported a past diagnosis of anorexia nervosa; however, 18 runners (14%) exceeded the EAT cutoff score indicative of disordered eating. The percentage of abnormal EAT scores was greatest for the elite ultramarathoners and collegiate cross-country runners and lowest for the recreational marathoners.
Wrestling			
Dale and Landers (1999)	85 junior high and high school wrestlers	EDI and EDE-Q	36% exceeded the EDI cutoff indicative of disordered eating during the in-season, while 19% exceeded the cutoff during the off-season. Only 2 wrestlers met the EDE-Q criteria for bulimia nervosa.

Lankin, Steen, and Oppliger (1990)	716 high school wrestlers	Questionnaire developed by the authors to evaluate bingeing, weight loss methods, and bulimic behaviors (using DSM-III criteria)	2.8% of wrestlers were diagnosed with bulimia nervosa based on DSM-III criteria. Wrestlers lost and regained an average of 2.5 kg/wk during the season. The most frequently used weight loss methods were increased exercise, food restriction, and dehydration using saunas.
Oppliger et al. (1993)	713 high school wrestlers	Questionnaire developed by the state of Wisconsin to assess weight loss practices and bulimic behaviors	1.7% met the DSM-III criteria for bulimia nervosa. 43% regularly practiced pathogenic weight control behaviors, including fasting (19%), fluid restriction (25%), rubber suits (34%), and self-induced vomiting (8%).
Steen and Brownell (1990)	63 collegiate and 368 high school wrestlers	Questionnaire developed by the authors to examine the frequency and magnitude of weight control methods and food preoccupation	41% of collegiate wrestlers reported weight fluctuations of 5-9 kg/wk; 23% of high school wrestlers lost 2.7-4.5 kg/wk. The most frequently used weight loss methods were food restriction (52%), fasting (26%), and dehydration (42%). Between 2% and 3% of all wrestlers used self-induced vomiting, diuretics, and laxatives once a week. 40% of all wrestlers reported being preoccupied with food and bingeing after a match.

(continued)

Table 2.1 *(continued)*

Study	Subjects	Instrument	Findings
Miscellaneous			
Beals 2002	123 elite male and female triathletes	A health, weight, dieting, and menstrual history questionnaire that included the EDI-DT and EDI-BD as well as self-reported history of ED	20% and 12.5% of the women reported a history of anorexia nervosa and bulimia nervosa, respectively. Both anorexia nervosa and bulimia nervosa were reported by 1.2% of the men. 15% of the men and 11% of the women reported they "might" have an eating disorder. 10% of the women and 5% of the men were "at risk" for an eating disorder based on EDI-DT scores, while 28% of the women and 8% of the men were at risk based on EDI-BD scores.
Dummer et al. (1987)	955 young swimmers (9-18 yr; 487 girls and 468 boys)	Michigan State University Weight Control Survey	15.4% of girls and 3.6% of boys reported using pathogenic weight control methods including self-induced vomiting (12.7% of girls and 2.7% of boys), diet pills (10.7% of girls and 6.8% of boys), laxatives (2.5% of girls and 4.1% of boys), and diuretics (1.5% of girls and 2.8% of boys).
King and Mezey (1987)	1 female and 13 male jockeys (19-35 yr)	EAT-26, Clinical Interview Schedule, semi-structured interview concerning eating and methods of weight control, Symptom Rating Test, Locus of Control Questionnaire	All jockeys reported regularly engaging in pathogenic weight control behaviors, including excessive exercise (100%), sauna (100%), rubber suits (86%), diuretics (43%), bingeing (43%), fasting (21%), appetite suppressants (14%), and self-induced vomiting (7%). However, none of the jockeys were diagnosed with a clinical eating disorder.

Marshall and Harber (1996)	111 female collegiate field hockey players	EDI	17.1% had EDI-BD and 3.6% had EDI-DT scores demonstrating eating disorder tendencies.
Olson et al. (1996)	30 female aerobic dance instructors	Biographical questionnaire and EDI	40% reported a history of disordered eating, 33% had elevated EDI-DT scores and 40% had elevated EDI-BD scores indicative of disordered eating.
Walberg and Johnston (1991)	103 female weight lifters	EDI and a self-developed instrument on training, menstruation, and dieting history	15.5% had elevated EDI-DT scores and 23.3% had elevated EDI-BD scores indicative of disordered eating. Many reported an exaggerated fear of fatness and obsession with food.

BULIT-R = Bulimia Test Revised (Thelen et al. 1991); EAT-26 = Eating Attitudes Test (26 questions; Garner et al. 1982); EAT-40 = Eating Attitudes Test (40 questions; Garner and Garfinkel 1979); EDI = Eating Disorder Inventory (Garner, Olmstead, and Polivy 1983); EDI-BD = Body Dissatisfaction subscale (Garner, Olmstead, and Polivy 1983); EDI-BUL = Bulimia subscale (Garner, Olmstead, and Polivy 1983); EDI-DT = Drive for Thinness subscale (Garner, Olmstead, and Polivy 1983); EDI-2 = Eating Disorder Inventory-2 (Garner 1991); EDE-Q = Eating Disorder Examination Questionnaire (Cooper and Fairburn 1987; Fairburn and Cooper 1993); Restrained Eating Scale (Stunkard 1981); BSQ = Body Shape Questionnaire (Cooper et al. 1987); Clinical Interview Schedule (CIS) (Goldberg et al. 1970); Eating interview (Szmkler 1983); Syptom-Rating test (Kellner and Sheffield 1973); Locus of Control Scale (Craig et al. 1984).

Methods of Assessing Eating Disorders

A final reason for the varying definitions of eating disorder used in prevalence studies is the diversity of screening instruments used. Only four studies in table 2.1 employed a clinical interview using the strict DSM-III or DSM-IV guidelines to identify eating disorders among athletes (Sundgot-Borgen 1993b; Le Grange, Tibbs, and Noakes 1994; Szmukler et al. 1985; Gadpille, Sanborn, and Wagner 1987). The remainder used self-report questionnaires such as the Eating Attitudes Test (EAT; Garner and Garfinkel 1979; Garner et al. 1982) or the Eating Disorder Inventory (EDI and EDI-2; Garner, Olmstead, and Polivy 1983; Garner 1991), surveys developed by the authors (of which many had not been previously tested for validity and reliability), or simply the frequency of disordered eating symptoms or pathogenic weight control behaviors (Beals and Manore 1999; Wilmore 1991). Again, the stricter the assessment criteria, the lower the prevalence is likely to be. Moreover, as is discussed at length in chapter 8, there is

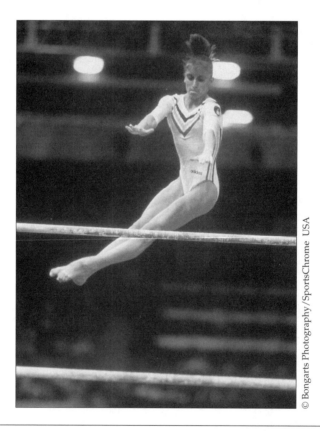

© Bongarts Photography/SportsChrome USA

Eating disorders are more prevalent among athletes in thin-build sports, including gymnastics.

considerable concern regarding the validity and reliability of self-report instruments for identifying athletes with eating disorders.

Despite the methodological inconsistencies and the resulting variations in prevalence estimates derived from the existing data, researchers generally concur that disordered eating poses a considerable threat to the health and well-being of a significant number of athletes. Moreover, most researchers maintain that the actual prevalence of disordered eating among athletes is apt to be higher than the figures presented in table 2.1, simply due to the fact that athletes likely underreport such disorders. Two studies reported in a review article by Wilmore (1991) support this contention.

In the first study reported by Wilmore (1991), the EAT was distributed to 110 elite female athletes representing seven different sports; 87 athletes completed and returned the survey. None of the athletes had elevated scores on the EAT (which indicate an eating disorder); during the two-year follow-up period, however, 18 of the athletes (16.4%) later received treatment for clinical eating disorders. In a second related study, 14 nationally ranked female distance runners completed the EDI. While just three runners initially had elevated EDI scores (indicative of possible disordered eating), seven were subsequently diagnosed with an eating disorder (four with anorexia nervosa, two with bulimia nervosa, and one with both).

These two studies suggest that, at least for female athletes, the use of self-report questionnaires to ascertain the prevalence of eating disorders may be invalid and thus may lead to a significant underestimation of the problem (Wilmore 1991). The idea that female athletes may be reluctant to self-report an eating disorder should come as no surprise. Admitting to an eating disorder is not akin to divulging one's true hair color or revealing one's actual age. Admitting to an eating disorder is acknowledging that one suffers from a serious psychological condition. For many people, particularly athletes, it is also acknowledging weakness and a loss of control. As described in chapter 1, individuals with eating disorders seek control above all else. In addition, they generally harbor feelings of guilt and shame regarding their disorder. They would be mortified if someone were to find out their secret! Moreover, athletes with eating disorders may fear discovery because of real and potentially serious repercussions, for example, being barred from competition, being removed from the team, or even losing an athletic scholarship.

A second reason that athletes are thought to be at a greater risk for disordered eating than nonathletes is athletes' characteristic personality traits. That is, athletes tend to be achievement driven, goal oriented, and perfectionistic, traits many consider vital to athletic success. Coincidentally, these very same traits are often seen in those with clinical eating disorders and are thought to contribute to the eating disorder "predisposition" (Sundgot-Borgen 1998). Thus, the athlete's personality may place him or her at a greater risk than a nonathlete for developing an eating disorder.

Another area of general agreement among researchers is that disordered eating is more prevalent among *female* athletes than *female* nonathletes

(Beals and Manore 1999; Brownell and Rodin 1992; Sundgot-Borgen 1998). A similar statement cannot be made for male athletes because of a lack of data. (This issue is discussed further in chapter 4.) At least three reasons for the greater prevalence of disordered eating among female athletes are hypothesized. First, female athletes are generally under greater pressure than their nonathletic counterparts to achieve and maintain a low body weight. They must conform not only to the general sociocultural ideal of slimness but also to the specific aesthetic or performance demands of their sport. For example, when the performance of a female gymnast or skater is judged, part of what the judges evaluate is the athlete's form and figure. For these sports in particular, the judges are looking for a petite, lithe body that glides effortlessly across the balance beam or the ice. Similarly, endurance athletes (e.g., cross-country runners and triathletes) often equate lower body weight with improvements in speed and economy of movement and thus enhanced performance (Beals and Manore 1999). Even sports that are not judged or are not thought to be significantly impacted by a reduction in body weight (sports such as volleyball, field hockey, swimming, tennis) often require that the athlete wear revealing clothing, which may trigger weight consciousness and subsequent disordered eating.

Timing may also help to explain the greater prevalence of disordered eating among athletes than among nonathletes. The onset of eating disorders in females typically occurs during late childhood or early adolescence. It is believed that emotional and physical changes that occur during adolescence increase vulnerability to eating disorders (APA 1994; Smolak et al. 1996). (This is discussed further in chapter 3.) Adolescence is also the time when many athletes reach the peak of their athletic careers and perhaps achieve elite status. The stress of training and competition and a win-at-all-costs attitude on top of the general stress associated with adolescence may render athletes more susceptible to disordered eating behaviors than nonathletes (Sundgot-Borgen 1998).

A final area of agreement among researchers is that disordered eating is more prevalent among athletes in sports that emphasize a low body weight or lean physique (i.e., thin-build sports) than those in which a low body weight is not considered advantageous (Beals and Manore 1999, 2002; Brownell and Rodin 1992; Smolak, Murnen, and Ruble 2000; Sundgot-Borgen 1993b, 1998; also see the sidebar). The two studies provide support for this notion.

What Are Thin-Build Sports, and Why Might They Foster a Higher Prevalence of Disordered Eating?

Thin-build sports, those in which a low body weight is thought to confer a competitive advantage, can be separated into three categories: (1) those that are judged (sometimes referred to as *aesthetic sports*), such as gymnastics, diving, figure skating, and dance (particularly ballet); (2) those in which a low body weight is thought to aid in the speed and efficiency of movement (generally endurance sports), such as distance running, cross-country skiing, and swimming; and (3) those that incorporate weight classifications, such as wrestling, powerlifting, bodybuilding, and karate, where failure to "make weight" means exclusion from competition.

Athletes participating in sports that are judged often feel pressure to conform to the low body weight and small body size ideals that are typically endorsed by the judges. Similarly, athletes participating in sports that require economy of movement may feel that weight loss will improve their speed, efficiency, and ultimately their endurance. Finally, athletes participating in sports with a weight classification are under pressure to make weight (and often attempt to diet down into a weight category below their natural weight for a presumed competitive advantage).

In the arguably most methodologically rigorous study of the prevalence of disordered eating to date, Sundgot-Borgen (1993b) examined disordered eating in a large sample of elite Norwegian female athletes (n = 522) representing 35 different sports. The sports were divided into two broad categories: (1) sports in which leanness or a specific weight were considered important (i.e., thin-build sports), including aesthetic, endurance, and weight-dependent sports, and (2) sports in which leanness or a specific weight were less important (i.e., non-thin-build sports), including technical, ball-game, and power sports. Athletes were screened for the clinical eating disorders anorexia and bulimia nervosa as well as a subclinical form of anorexia (anorexia athletica) using a combination of self-report questionnaires, a physical examination, and a clinical interview based on the DSM-III diagnostic criteria. The results indicated that both clinical and subclinical eating disorders were significantly more prevalent among athletes in thin-build sports (particularly aesthetic and weight-dependent sports) than among those in non-thin-build sports.

In a similar study, Beals and Manore (2002) examined the prevalence of disordered eating in female collegiate athletes (n = 425) representing seven different sports. The sports were categorized into aesthetic sports (cheerleading, diving, gymnastics), endurance sports (basketball, cross-country and track [middle-distance and distance events], field hockey, crew, soccer, swimming, and water polo), and anaerobic team sports (track [field events], golf, softball, tennis, and volleyball). Disordered eating was assessed by a weight and dieting history questionnaire, the 26-item Eating Attitudes Test (EAT-26), and the Eating Disorder Inventory Body Dissatisfaction subscale (EDI-BD). A similar percentage of athletes in aesthetic, endurance, and anaerobic sports reported a clinical diagnosis of anorexia nervosa (5.6%, 3.5%, and 1.0%, respectively). Neither were there significant differences in the percentages of athletes in aesthetic, endurance, and anaerobic sports who reported a clinical diagnosis of bulimia nervosa (5.6%, 1.6%, and 2.1%, respectively). However, athletes in aesthetic sports scored significantly higher on the EAT-26 (13.5 ± 10.9) than athletes in endurance

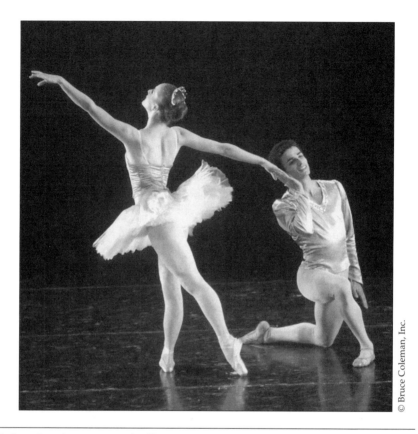

© Bruce Coleman, Inc.

Eating disorders pose a significant threat to the health and well-being of far too many athletes, particularly those in thin-build sports.

(10.0 ± 9.3) or anaerobic sports (9.9 ± 9.0). In addition, significantly more athletes in aesthetic than in endurance or anaerobic sports scored above the EAT-26 cutoff score of 20, indicating that they demonstrated behaviors characteristic of those with an eating disorder.

Even though researchers cannot agree on a specific value for the prevalence of disordered eating among athletes, they generally agree that the prevalence is higher than it should be. Most also agree that prevalence figures currently available underestimate the true prevalence of disordered eating among athletes, particularly among female athletes and especially among those in thin-build sports.

Summary

The prevalence of disordered eating among female athletes has been reported to be as low as 1% and as high as 62%, while the prevalence among male athletes lies somewhere between 0% and 57%. These wide-ranging estimates are due to differences in screening instruments used, definitions of eating disorders employed, and athletic populations studied. Nonetheless, despite the conflicting prevalence estimates derived from the available research, it is generally agreed that eating disorders pose a significant threat to the health and well-being of far too many athletes, particularly female athletes participating in thin-build sports. Moreover, the shame and potentially serious repercussions of discovery may contribute to underreporting by athletes and thus general underestimation of the prevalence of disordered eating in sports.

three

Etiology of Disordered Eating in Athletes

CHAPTER OBJECTIVES

After reading this chapter, you will be able to

- identify the risk factors for the development of disordered eating and

- identify the factors inherent in or unique to the athletic environment that may place athletes at risk for disordered eating.

Why do some athletes develop eating disorders, while others remain relatively immune? This question has plagued researchers and practitioners for decades. Currently there is no definitive answer; rather, most eating disorder experts maintain that many factors independently or collectively place an athlete at risk for developing an eating disorder.

An equally daunting question, one that has fueled heated debate among eating disorder specialists, is whether athletes are at a greater risk of developing disordered eating behaviors than their nonathletic counterparts. It is a debate that is likely to continue for some time because few studies have directly compared athletes with nonathletes in terms of eating disorder incidence, and the results of these studies are equivocal (Byrne and McLean 2001; Davis 1990; Davis and Cowles 1989; Smolak, Murnen, and Ruble 2000; Sundgot-Borgen 1993b, 1994; Borgen and Corbin 1987; Tiggemann and Pickering 1996; Williamson et al. 1995). For example, Taub and Blinde (1992) found that adolescent athletes competing in a variety of sports were more likely than nonathletes to possess certain behavioral and psychological traits associated with disordered eating. Similarly, in a study examining the prevalence of disordered eating among elite Norwegian athletes, Sundgot-Borgen (1993b) found that a significantly higher percentage of athletes than nonathletic controls met the diagnostic criteria for anorexia and bulimia nervosa. In sharp contrast to these studies, Borgen and Corbin (1987) found no overall difference in the prevalence of disordered eating between collegiate athletes and nonathletes. It should be noted, however, that when the athletes were separated based on the degree to which their sport emphasized a low body weight, it was found that athletes in the thin-build sports were more likely to demonstrate disordered eating behaviors than either nonathletes or athletes participating in sports that did not emphasize a low body weight.

This chapter explores hypothesized causes of disordered eating in athletes and examines the circumstances or factors unique to the athletic environment that may place the athlete at increased risk of developing disordered eating.

Risk Factors for the Development of Disordered Eating

Most eating disorder specialists agree that the etiology of disordered eating in both athletes and nonathletes is multifactorial and includes a complex interaction between sociocultural, demographic, environmental, biological, psychological, and behavioral factors.

Sociocultural Factors

Eating disorders are significantly more prevalent in industrialized and Westernized countries (e.g., Australia, Canada, England, France, and the

United States) than in nonindustrialized or less-industrialized countries. The reason for this cultural difference is not completely understood but is thought to be due to the various societal influences that are unique to Westernized countries (Rodin and Larson 1992; Wiseman et al. 1992), one of the most pervasive being attitudes about body weight. In most modern Westernized societies, being thin is equated with beauty, as well as a number of other positive attributes, including goodness, success, and power (Rodin 1993).

Women in particular are led to believe that they must be thin in order to be accepted by society. This belief is both reinforced and perpetuated by the images presented in movies, television, and magazines (Garner and Garfinkel 1980; Thompson and Sherman 1993; Wilkens, Boland, and Albinson 1991). The emaciated figures gracing the covers and filling the pages of popular women's magazines have been blamed for the increased prevalence of weight obsession and disordered eating (Field et al. 1999; Garner and Garfinkel 1980; Harrison and Cantor 1997; Rodin 1993; Thompson and Sherman 1993; Wilkens, Boland, and Albinson 1991). For example, a recent study showed that reading popular women's magazines (e.g., *Shape, Cosmopolitan, Vogue*) known to contain numerous pictures of extremely thin models as well as articles on dieting was the most consistent predictor of disordered eating symptoms among young women when compared with other forms of mass media exposure (Harrison and Cantor 1997). Similarly, television viewing has been associated with the development of disordered eating, although total viewing time is thought to be less important than the type of programs watched. Interestingly, daytime and nighttime soap operas were most positively associated with eating disorder symptoms (Tiggemann and Pickering 1996).

Although women experience the brunt of societal pressure to be thin, men are beginning to succumb to body weight and shape pressures with increasing frequency. Little formal research has been done, but indirect evidence and anecdotal reports suggest that men, particularly those engaged in athletics or who are regularly physically active, are becoming increasingly concerned and subsequently dissatisfied with their bodies (Pope, Phillips, and Olivardia 2000). (This is discussed further in chapter 4.)

It has been suggested that athletes face even greater pressure than nonathletes to achieve or maintain a particular body weight or shape (Sundgot-Borgen 1994). As described in chapter 2, athletes must not only meet the current body weight ideals held by society in general but also conform to the specific aesthetic and performance demands of their sport. This pressure may be particularly high for athletes in thin-build sports or activities that require a low body weight or lean physique, such as dance (especially ballet), gymnastics, distance running, triathlon, swimming, diving, figure skating, cheerleading, wrestling, and lightweight rowing. Research confirms that female athletes frequently feel pressure from coaches or teammates to achieve or maintain a particular body weight and cite this pressure as an impetus for the development of pathogenic weight control behaviors (Beals and Manore 2000; Garner, Rosen, and Barry 1998; Sundgot-Borgen 1993a, 1993b). Although little formal research has been done with male subjects, the popularity of men's muscle and fitness magazines seems to indicate that men are not completely free from pressure to achieve a particular body weight or shape.

This pressure can be particularly strong (rendering the development of an eating disorder much more likely) when there is a discrepancy between the athlete's actual body weight and the perceived ideal body weight for the athlete's chosen sport (Brownell and Rodin 1992). For example, a naturally larger athlete who wishes to compete in gymnastics or a naturally heavier wrestler who is trying to compete in a lower weight class may feel especially strong pressure to alter his or her body weight.

Psychosocial Factors

Individuals who develop eating disorders often come from dysfunctional families, particularly those involving overbearing or controlling parents, physical or sexual abuse, or parental alcoholism or substance abuse (Brownell and Foryet 1986; Fairburn et al. 1997). Such familial environments can cause severe psychological and emotional distress, undermine the development of self-esteem, and lead to inadequate coping skills, all of which may place an individual at an increased risk for developing an eating disorder. For example, a psychologically vulnerable individual who lacks the coping skills to handle a stressful situation may focus his or her energies on controlling body weight as a means of establishing a sense of control over a chaotic family life. Although this may not be a common causative factor in athletes, it should always be considered a possibility. For example, an athlete may feel overwhelmed or out of control as a result of an injury, a particularly poor performance, or the excessive demands of a coach. Because of a dysfunctional family environment, the athlete may have never developed the coping skills necessary to handle these problems, and thus the athlete concentrates on something that can be managed, such as body weight.

Granted, not all dysfunctional families produce children with disordered eating. Nonetheless, the familial characteristics just described can certainly set the stage for the development of disordered eating, particularly in those with a psychological predisposition. It has been hypothesized that individuals who are perfectionistic, achievement oriented, independent, persistent, and tolerant of pain and discomfort and who have high self-expectations yet low self-esteem are more susceptible to the development of disordered eating (Garfinkel, Garner, and Goldbloom 1987).

Coincidentally, many of these same personality traits are characteristic of the competitive athlete. In fact, as previously mentioned, these personality traits are considered key to success in sports, which may help explain the increased risk of eating disorders among athletes, particularly elite athletes (Garner, Rosen, and Barry 1998). Indeed, it is not difficult to understand how an athlete who seeks perfection in all things (including body weight), who is goal oriented and driven to excel, and who is capable of and often programmed to tolerate pain (i.e., to "suck it up") can readily succumb to an eating disorder. Just as athletes push their bodies to physical limits to achieve a high level of performance, so too can athletes push themselves to achieve or maintain a low body weight, despite potential negative consequences to performance or health.

Demographic Factors

Prevalence data clearly indicate that eating disorders are more common among certain segments of the population. What the data do not definitively indicate is whether certain demographic characteristics predispose an individual to developing disordered eating (i.e., whether there is a cause-and-effect relationship) or whether the relationship is merely an association. The demographic characteristics that have been shown to be related to disordered eating include gender, age, and ethnicity.

Gender

With women outnumbering men 10:1 in eating disorder prevalence, gender is considered one of the primary demographic determinants of susceptibility to disordered eating (APA 1994; Garner, Rosen, and Barry 1998). Although few studies have directly compared eating disorder prevalence between female and male athletes, the limited data suggest that female athletes are at greater risk than their male counterparts (Johnson, Powers, and Dick 1999; Sundgot-Borgen 1999). This disordered eating gender gap is thought to be caused by a number of factors, including the disparity in sociocultural expectations regarding body weight (see the previous section on sociocultural factors) as well as biological, hormonal, and evolutionary differences between the sexes. An additional factor that may explain the increased susceptibility of female athletes to disordered eating is the increased focus on the female athlete's body weight and shape. Indeed, it is rare to hear a sportscaster comment on the body weight of a male figure skater, gymnast, or tennis player; however, body weights of female athletes seem to be a frequent topic of conversation among sports commentators (particularly if there has been a recent weight gain).

Age

Although eating disorders can occur at any time in life, they typically begin in adolescence, with anorexia nervosa often developing somewhat earlier than bulimia nervosa (APA 1994). Adolescence is a particularly vulnerable period both physically and psychologically, a time when the body is going through enormous change. For girls especially, the physiological changes that accompany growing into womanhood (e.g., the increase in body fat, breast and hip development) can cause significant distress. Moreover, the body weight and shape changes that occur as a young girl goes through puberty generally take her further away from the current ideal body shape; thus, she may begin to diet or engage in disordered eating behaviors to try to maintain a prepubescent weight and shape. Conversely, even though boys' physiological changes are no less significant, they generally do not cause the same degree of distress to boys as to girls. As boys develop into men, they tend to gain body weight and experience increases in muscular size and strength. Thus, unlike girls, as boys mature, they get ever closer to the ideal male body weight and shape.

In addition to the physical transformation, significant psychological and emotional changes occur during adolescence. Most adolescents are struggling to solidify their sense of self and develop their psychological and emotional independence. They may use weight management as a means of managing the emotional chaos of puberty (APA 1994).

Age also appears to play a role in the development of disordered eating among athletes. Research suggests that athletes who begin sport training at an early age are at increased risk of developing disordered eating (Sundgot-Borgen 1994). There are at least two possible explanations for this phenomenon. It may be that athletes who begin training for their sport early in

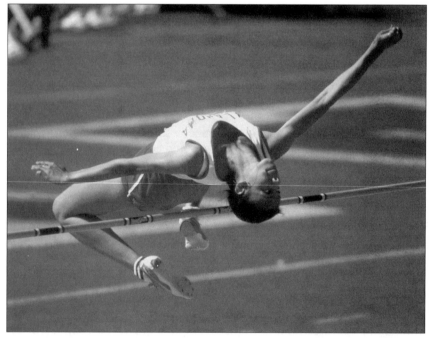

© Dave Johnson/Bruce Coleman, Inc.

Sports in which a low weight or body fat percentage is thought to confer a physiological advantage (e.g., distance running, high jump) may place athletes at greater risk for developing disordered eating.

life (i.e., before they have developed and matured) are less able to choose a sport that matches their body size, weight, or shape than those who begin training later in life (i.e., after they have developed and matured). Research indicates that the more an athlete's body weight or shape deviates from the ideal of his or her sport, the greater the risk of developing disordered eating (Brownell and Rodin 1992). It may also be that the athlete who begins sport-specific training at an early age or who has been involved in training for many years has no concept of self outside the athletic realm. As detailed in chapter 1, often an athlete's sense of self-worth is determined by athletic performance. Anything that threatens athletic performance threatens the athlete's very sense of self. In the face of such threats, adolescent athletes might be willing to go to extremes (including pathogenically controlling their weight) to protect their athletic identity (Taub and Blinde 1992).

For example, the young female gymnast who begins training and experiences athletic success at a young age will be significantly distressed (and her performance will likely decline) when her body begins to develop and mature (and she begins to gain weight and body fat). She may attempt to delay or prevent this development (and the accompanying weight gain) with stringent dieting and excessive exercise, which could ultimately lead to disordered eating behaviors. This scenario is most frequently seen in sports where early sport-specific training is common (e.g., gymnastics, figure skating, swimming).

Ethnicity

Research consistently indicates that, among the general public, the prevalence of clinical eating disorders among nonwhite ethnic groups is significantly lower than among whites (Garner and Garfinkel 1980; Hsu 1990). This difference is thought to be due to differences in cultural expectations regarding body weight, socioeconomic dynamics, and biological factors. Based on the low incidence of disordered eating among nonwhite ethnic groups in the general population, one would expect a similarly low incidence among nonwhite athletes. Surprisingly, very few studies have examined the prevalence of disordered eating among nonwhite athletes, and the existing studies suffer methodological flaws that make it difficult to derive definitive conclusions. The most significant methodological weakness among these studies is the underrepresentation (albeit largely unintentional) of nonwhite athletes in the subject samples (Taub and Blinde 1992). To be sure, the sports that are generally targeted when examining eating disorder prevalence (and which have been shown to have a high prevalence of disordered eating) are those in which participation of nonwhite athletes is generally low (e.g., gymnastics, diving, figure skating, cross-country running, swimming). Thus, these samples are ethnically biased at the outset and may serve to skew eating disorder prevalence estimates among nonwhite athletes.

An unpublished manuscript described by Thompson and Sherman (1993), in their book *Helping Athletes With Eating Disorders*, supports this notion. The authors examined team membership and disordered eating risk factors among nonwhite female collegiate athletes and found a trend toward an "inverse relationship between the percentage of black athletes on a given team and the mean number of eating disorder risk factors for each athlete on that team" (Thompson and Sherman 1993, p. 24). In other words, the more black athletes on a team, the fewer eating disorder risk factors. This statistic by itself might lead us to conclude that black athletes *are* at a lower risk for eating disorders than their white counterparts. However, the authors also noted that very few black athletes (just under 8%) participated in what are considered high-risk sports (e.g., gymnastics, cross-country running, diving), while the majority were found in the low-risk sports of basketball (54.5%) and track (56.3%). According to Thompson and Sherman, this underrepresentation of nonwhite athletes in high-risk sports is not confined to this particular study; similar participation percentages have been reported in surveys of NCAA member institutions (Thompson and Sherman 1993, p. 24).

It is quite likely that the lower reported incidence of disordered eating among nonwhite athletes is simply due to sampling bias. Alternatively, it could be that nonwhite athletes do not develop disordered eating as frequently as their white counterparts because they do not often participate in high-risk sports and thus are less apt to be exposed to the body weight and shape pressures posed by these sports.

Biological Factors

Some researchers have postulated that imbalances in various hormones and neurotransmitters may predispose certain individuals to developing disordered eating behaviors (Goldbloom and Garfinkel 1990; Kaye and Weltzin 1991; Kennedy 1994). *Serotonin,* a neurotransmitter that plays a significant role in hunger and satiety, has probably received the most attention from researchers for its potential role in the development or maintenance of eating disorders, particularly bulimia nervosa (Goldbloom and Garfinkel 1990; Kaye and Weltzin 1991). According to the *serotonin hypothesis,* bulimia nervosa is the behavioral expression of decreased levels or activity of serotonin in the central nervous system (Goldbloom and Garfinkel 1990). Research has shown that decreased brain levels of serotonin can to lead to increased carbohydrate intake and impairment of satiety (Goldbloom and Garfinkel 1990). The binge of the bulimic patient is similarly characterized by the consumption of large amounts of carbohydrate and a blunted satiety response. Theoretically then, the bulimic binge could be a response to decreased levels of serotonin in the brain.

Not only do neurotransmitters regulate eating behavior, but diet in turn can affect neurotransmitter synthesis and activity. Moreover, these effects may be somewhat gender specific, which may help to explain why women outnumber men in disordered eating. For example, in a study examining the differential effects of energy restriction on hypothalamic serotonin levels in men and women, it was found that just three weeks of energy restriction

(1,000 kcal/d for women and 1,200 kcal/d for men) significantly decreased serotonin activity in women but not men (Kaye and Weltzin 1991).

Melatonin has also been linked to disordered eating behavior, although its etiological and clinical significance are currently unknown (Kennedy 1994). A hormone that is produced by the body in the greatest quantities at night, melatonin is associated with a decrease in body temperature and feelings of sleepiness. Because serotonin is a precursor of melatonin, changes in serotonin levels (as have been demonstrated in both anorexic and bulimic patients) could also theoretically affect melatonin levels. Moreover, individuals who suffer from seasonal affective disorder (SAD, which is characterized by elevated daytime levels of serotonin and subsequently melatonin) demonstrate similar symptoms to those with bulimia, such as fatigue, carbohydrate cravings, and unexplained weight gain (Kennedy 1994). Research in animals as well as some limited research in humans has demonstrated that energy restriction can lead to elevated daytime levels of melatonin (Kennedy 1994). Thus, alterations in melatonin levels could help to explain the carbohydrate cravings characteristic of individuals suffering from bulimia nervosa.

A biological-behavioral model of activity-based anorexia nervosa was proposed in a series of studies by Epling and Pierce (1988) and Epling, Pierce, and Stefan (1993). These researchers theorized that strenuous exercise suppresses appetite, which leads to decreased food intake and subsequent reduction in body weight (and thus may initiate the anorexic cycle). It should be noted that this research was conducted with rats and has not been replicated in humans (O'Connor and Smith 1999). Additional biological factors that have been implicated in the development of disordered eating include early onset of menarche (<12 yr) and a propensity toward obesity (APA 1994; Fairburn et al. 1997).

Sport-Specific Factors

Recent research findings indicate that certain pressures or demands inherent in the sport setting may trigger the development of an eating disorder in psychologically susceptible athletes (Sundgot-Borgen 1994; Taub and Blinde 1992; Webb and Puig-Domingo 1995). For example, in a study investigating the prevalence of eating disorders in elite female athletes, Sundgot-Borgen (1994) found that pressures regarding body size and shape characteristic of aesthetic and weight-dependent sports were influential in the development of eating disorders. Specific trigger factors that appeared to put the athlete at risk of developing an eating disorder included the following:

■ Prolonged periods of dieting or weight cycling. Athletes often feel pressure to lose weight rapidly in order to make weight or meet a weight standard set by the coach. Such athletes are more likely to engage in pathogenic forms of weight loss and *weight cycling* (cycles of losing and regaining weight), behaviors that have been shown to precede the development of eating disorders in athletes.

■ Sudden increases in training volume. Some endurance athletes have reported that their eating disorder developed subsequent to a sudden and significant increase in their training load. These reports are supported by a study by Costill (1988), who found that athletes who increased their training volume experienced a decrease in appetite that resulted in weight loss. Similarly, data from a study by Brownell and Rodin (1992) indicated that training intensity was positively correlated to the development of eating disorders in male runners.

■ Stress and trauma. Stressful situations and traumatic events (e.g., injury, illness, change or loss of a coach, moving away from friends and family) have been associated with the development of disordered eating behaviors in susceptible athletes (Sundgot-Borgen 1994). It has been hypothesized that these traumatic events leave the athlete feeling vulnerable and out of control. Thus, the athlete may attempt to manage body weight to reestablish a sense of control. Similarly, an injury or illness that leaves the athlete unable to train for a prolonged period of time may cause him or her to feel helpless and vulnerable. Feeling out of control and concerned about weight gain during the training lapse, the athlete may develop increasingly restrictive eating behaviors or pathogenic weight control techniques that may eventually develop into an eating disorder.

■ Pressure from coaches and trainers. A number of studies have reported that athletes started dieting stringently after a coach advised them to lose weight (Rosen and Hough 1988; Sundgot-Borgen 1994). For example, Rosen and Hough (1988) found that 75% of athletes who were told by their coaches that they were too heavy started using pathogenic weight control methods. Recent research, however, suggests that it may not be the directive to lose weight that is problematic but rather the lack of guidance during the weight loss that predisposes an athlete to disordered eating. For example, Sundgot-Borgen (1994) found that among athletes who had been told by a coach to diet but did not develop an eating disorder, most (75%) had received guidance during their weight loss. In contrast, 90% of athletes who did develop eating disorders received no guidance on proper weight loss. Unfortunately, most studies indicate that coaches lack the nutritional knowledge necessary to provide sound nutritional advice and guidance regarding weight loss to their athletes (Parr, Porter, and Hodgson 1984).

Some researchers have proposed that specific sports or physical activities (i.e., those that emphasize leanness or require large training volumes) may attract individuals with eating disorders, particularly anorexia nervosa, because it provides them with a setting in which they can hide or justify their abnormal eating and dieting behaviors (Sacks 1990). Endurance sports and sports that require large amounts of aerobic exercise may attract individuals with disordered eating since they can use (or abuse) exercise to expend extra calories and keep body weight low. The stereotyped standards of body shape in women's sports and physical activities that emphasize leanness also make it difficult for observers to notice when an athlete has

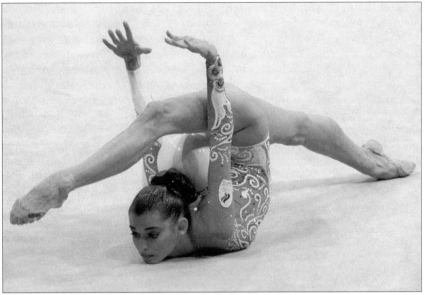

© Empics

Pressure to be thin can be particularly strong when an athlete does not conform to the perceived ideal body weight for a particular sport. This pressure increases the likelihood that the athlete will develop an eating disorder.

lost too much weight. These common and accepted low weight standards may help active women with disordered eating hide or justify their problem and delay intervention (Sacks 1990; Sundgot-Borgen 1993b).

Summary

Certain inherent aspects of the athletic environment may increase an athlete's risk for developing disordered eating behaviors. The pressure to achieve or maintain a low body weight or body fat percentage can stem from an external source (e.g., coach, trainer, teammates) or internally from the athlete herself or himself. The sport setting naturally imposes heightened body awareness on the athlete, particularly the female athlete who often is required to wear revealing uniforms. In an attempt to meet the aesthetic demands of their sport and/or improve performance, athletes may engage in inappropriate dieting and weight loss behaviors that may eventually progress into a full-blown eating disorder (particularly if they do not receive guidance in their weight loss).

The personality characteristics common among athletes may also make them more susceptible to disordered eating. Perfectionism, compulsiveness, and being goal oriented are all personality traits that are instrumental to athletic success. Unfortunately, they are the same personality traits frequently displayed by those with clinical eating disorders. Athletes are also known for their mental strength and focus. To be successful, they must learn to block distraction and even pain when they train. Thus, they may also be able to block hunger and other feelings that accompany severe energy restriction and disordered eating. Finally, many athletes are motivated to win at all costs. At high levels of competition, the stakes are high (e.g., achieving or maintaining a scholarship or sponsorship, winning a gold medal), and the possibility is greater that the athlete is willing to take unnecessary risks to win.

Although disordered eating has been identified in a wide range of sports, some sports place athletes at higher risk of the development of these behaviors, including sports in which subjective judging encourages a small, lean appearance (e.g., gymnastics, dance, figure skating, diving), sports in which a low body weight is thought to confer a physiological advantage (e.g., distance running, jumping, cross-country skiing, triathlon), and sports with weight classifications (e.g., weightlifting, wrestling, rowing, martial arts).

four

Disordered Eating in Male Athletes

CHAPTER OBJECTIVES

After reading this chapter, you will be able to

■ describe the prevalence of disordered eating in male athletes,

■ explain the reasons for the higher prevalence of disordered eating in female athletes than in male athletes (i.e., the eating disorder gender gap),

■ identify the similarities and differences between male and female athletes with eating disorders, and

■ describe muscle dysmorphia, also known as the "Adonis complex."

Eating Disorders and the Male Experience

Although weight issues have plagued men for centuries, their plight has been largely eclipsed by the greater attention given to weight and eating disturbances in women. A review of the literature spanning the 17th to 19th centuries reveals several published reports of self-starvation in young males. In fact, the first published medical description of anorexia nervosa (in 1694) documented *both* a female and a male case (Mickalide 1990).

Despite the acknowledgment that men can and do develop eating disorders, the general belief remains that eating disorders in males are so rare as to be of little clinical significance. To be sure, the incidence of eating disorders in males is relatively low (0.01%-0.04% of the population), and with a prevalence ratio of 10:1 (female to male cases) is considered significantly lower than that reported for females, (APA 1994). Nonetheless, disordered eating in males is far from insignificant, as this chapter will demonstrate.

Like male nonathletes with eating disorders, male athletes with eating disorders are considered a rarity, their numbers insignificant compared with their female counterparts. While exact prevalence figures are currently unknown, most researchers speculate that the prevalence in athletes follows a pattern similar to that of nonathletes, such that female athletes with disordered eating significantly outnumber male athletes. A few researchers and practitioners, however, believe that current prevalence figures underestimate the true incidence of disordered eating among males, particularly male athletes (Andersen 1992, 2001). One of these researchers is Harrison Pope, lead author of *The Adonis Complex: The Secret Crisis of Male Body Obsession* (Pope, Phillips, and Olivardia 2000). According to Pope, "Millions of boys and men today harbor a secret obsession about their looks and are endangering their health by engaging in excessive exercise, bingeing and purging rituals, steroid abuse, and overuse of nutritional and dietary supplements" (Pope, Phillips, and Olivardia 2000).

A quick perusal of men's magazines along with a glance inside the local gym supports the notion that men are becoming increasingly concerned about their bodies and are working hard to improve them. But is this growing interest in body weight and fitness among males evidence of increasing prevalence of eating disorders, and more important, can it really be compared with the body image disturbances and eating disorders suffered more traditionally by women?

This chapter examines disordered eating in male athletes through comparisons with disordered eating in female athletes. Specifically, similarities and differences between eating disorders in male and female athletes in prevalence, etiology, and disease progression are discussed. The recently identified body image disorder described in male athletes known as *muscle dysmorphia* or the "Adonis complex" is also described.

Prevalence of Disordered Eating
in Male Compared to Female Athletes

Few studies have directly compared eating disorder prevalence between male and female athletes participating in a wide variety of sports. Nonetheless, it would be expected that disordered eating would be less common among male than female athletes because both epidemiological research and clinical case studies consistently demonstrate a higher prevalence of eating disorders among women than men (Garner, Rosen, and Barry 1998). The limited existing research comparing disordered eating in male and female athletes seems to support this presumption (Johnson, Powers, and Dick 1999; Petrie 1996; Sundgot-Borgen et al. 1999; Sykora et al. 1993).

In the largest U.S. survey to date, Johnson, Powers, and Dick (1999) examined the prevalence of disordered eating among 883 male and 562 female athletes from 11 NCAA Division I schools and competing in a variety of sports. A 133-item questionnaire developed by the authors was used to identify four eating disorder categories: (1) clinically diagnosable eating disorder (based on the DSM-IV criteria), (2) self-identified eating disorder, (3) subclinical eating disorder, (4) "at risk" for an eating disorder. As might be expected, the prevalence of disordered eating among women exceeded that of men. Slightly over 1% of the female athletes met the diagnostic criteria for a clinical eating disorder, while 12% presented with a subclinical eating disorder. In contrast, none of the male athletes met the diagnostic criteria for a clinical eating disorder and only 0.01% presented with a subclinical eating disorder. Additionally, the percentages of athletes considered to be "at risk for" anorexia and bulimia nervosa was significantly greater for women (35% and 58%, respectively) than for men (9.5% and 38%, respectively).

In a similar study, Sundgot-Borgen et al. (1999) examined the prevalence of eating disorders in elite male ($n = 960$) and female ($n = 660$) Norwegian athletes representing 60 different sporting events. Using a dieting questionnaire that included subscales of the EDI and a self-reported history of eating disorders, the researchers found that the prevalence of disordered eating (namely anorexia nervosa, bulimia nervosa, and EDNOS) was significantly higher for female (20%) than male (8%) athletes.

Taking a somewhat different approach, Dick (1991) surveyed athletic administrators from 491 NCAA member institutions to determine the incidence of eating disorders in both men's and women's sports over a two-year period (1988-1990). Unlike other prevalence studies, this study did not seek to determine the total number of eating disorder cases, but rather whether at least one case had been reported and, if so, in which sport or sports they had occurred. Three hundred and thirteen institutions (64%) indicated that at least one student athlete had an eating disorder. In all, 810 eating disorder cases were reported from women's sports versus just 62 from men's sports. It should be noted that these "incidence" figures likely represent an underestimation of eating disorder prevalence, as it is highly probable that more than one case occurred within a given sport. Nonetheless, the data clearly show that eating disorders occur less frequently in men's than in women's sports.

Eating Disorder Gender Gap

The reasons for the higher eating disorder prevalence among female than male athletes are not completely understood but are hypothesized to be rooted in the different sociocultural expectations and sport-specific demands placed on females and males. As described in chapter 3, researchers consistently implicate the overwhelming sociocultural pressure to be thin (and the social stigmatization of overweight and obesity) as a key determinant in the etiology of eating disorders (Garner and Garfinkel 1980; Rodin 1993). Because women are typically judged more by their appearance than men, greater emphasis is placed on a women's body weight and shape, and thus women tend to be at increased risk of developing body image disturbances and subsequent disordered eating behaviors.

Female athletes, like their nonathletic counterparts, are also more apt to be judged along aesthetic lines than male athletes; thus, body weight and shape are apt to play a greater role in the evaluation of the female athlete's performance. This is particularly true in sports that are judged, such as gymnastics, figure skating, cheerleading, and diving, where form and figure play a large part in the way in which the athlete's performance is evaluated. Sports in which a low weight or body fat percentage is thought to confer a physiological advantage (e.g., distance running, sprinting, long jump, high jump) may also place the female athlete at greater risk of disordered eating than her male counterpart. Because men naturally have less body fat and more lean body mass as well as a higher metabolic rate (largely due to their greater lean body mass) than women, they are less likely to have to diet to achieve the body weight or composition deemed necessary for success in their sport. Even in sports in which a low body weight or body fat percentage is not considered aesthetically or physiologically advantageous (e.g., swimming, volleyball, tennis), there seems to be greater pressure on women to slim down just for the sake of looking good in their uniforms (Slear 2001).

This notion is supported by Selby et al. (1990), who compared body image and weight control behaviors in male (n = 138) and female (n = 109) collegiate athletes representing 27 sport teams. The researchers found that significantly more female than male athletes felt that weight was "critical" to performance. In addition, significantly more women than men reported difficulty in attaining and maintaining both their own ideal competitive weight and the weight suggested by their coach. Finally, female athletes experienced more negative emotional responses (i.e., anger, anxiety, frustration, and depression) when they were unable to reach or maintain their ideal weight.

While gender-related differences in sport-specific demands regarding body weight or composition are no doubt a contributing factor to the disordered eating gender gap, we cannot discount the possibility that the disparity between male and female athletes in eating disorder prevalence is due to underreporting. Andersen (1992) has suggested that, for a variety of reasons, cases of male athletes with eating disorders are underreported and that the statistical scarcity of such disorders in males may make it more difficult for clinicians to recognize them when they do occur. Part of this difficulty lies in the cultural bias of viewing disordered eating as a "woman's disease" (Andersen and Holman 1997). People do not typically associate eating disorders with men. Thus, what would be clearly identifiable eating disorder symptoms in a woman are often overlooked or completely ignored in a man. For example, an emaciated man is likely viewed as thin or skinny, whereas an equally emaciated woman might be labeled "anorexic." Similarly, a man who consumes large portions of food rapidly or who engages in excessive exercise might be described as having a "healthy appetite" and even admired for his dedication to fitness or his sport. A woman demonstrating the same behaviors would be called "bulimic" and a "compulsive exerciser." These same gender stereotypes likely hold true for male and female athletes.

The labeling of an eating disorder as a "woman's disease" may also render males more reluctant to present themselves for treatment, as they may be embarrassed to admit to having a woman's problem or think they can or should handle the problem themselves. The embarrassment associated with disclosure likely contributes to underreporting in males and biases prevalence estimates. Finally, Andersen (1992) contends that subtle but significant developmental and behavioral differences between male and female athletes with eating disorders make recognizing disordered eating in male athletes slightly more complex.

Comparison of Male and Female Athletes With Disordered Eating

Key to understanding, identifying, and managing disordered eating in male athletes is recognizing the similarities and differences between the genders when it comes to eating disorders. The following sections compare and contrast disordered eating in males and females along developmental, behavioral, and physiological lines. Because there is so little data specific to athletes, the focus is on the current state of knowledge in nonathletes and how that might translate to athletes.

Similarities

Most researchers and practitioners maintain that disordered eating in males is more similar than dissimilar to that in females. Moreover, as the severity of the eating disorder increases, so too do the similarities (Andersen 1992).

Because of the dearth of research in the area of sex differences (and similarities) in disordered eating in athletes, we can only assume that those seen in nonathletes hold true for athletes as well.

Predisposition

Research indicates that both males and females with disordered eating have a high probability of coming from families with affective disorders or having a personal history of mood or personality disorders (Andersen 1992). In addition, both male and females with disordered eating demonstrate similar personality traits (i.e., perfectionism, goal orientation, high self-expectation, drive to achieve, and introversion), traits that are believed to make them more psychologically vulnerable to the development of disordered eating. Finally, both males and females who develop disordered eating tend to belong to societal subgroups that encourage a reduction in body weight or a lean body composition (Sundgot-Borgen et al. 1999).

In the case of male and female athletes, disordered eating behaviors tend to develop most frequently in those who participate in thin-build sports (Andersen 1992; Brownell and Rodin 1992). As described in chapter 2, thin-build sports include aesthetic sports, endurance sports, and sports that employ weight classifications. For male athletes, eating disorder risk appears to be particularly high in sports that employ weight classifications, including wrestling, rowing, bodybuilding, and horse racing (Blouin and Goldfield 1995; Pasman and Thompson 1988; Steen and Brownell 1990; Sykora et al. 1993).

Wrestlers are the male athletes most often identified as a population at risk for eating disorders. In the surveillance study that examined eating disorders in NCAA athletic programs, Dick (1991) found that of the 67 (out of 801) schools reporting an eating disorder in a particular sport, 20 involved wrestling. Wrestlers often cut weight to compete in weight classes that are 15 lb (6.8 kg) or more below their off-season weight, believing that this will afford them a competitive advantage over naturally smaller opponents (American College of Sports Medicine 1996). Unfortunately, weight cutting is often done quickly (in a matter of days or sometimes hours), using dangerous or pathogenic methods. In a study of 125 high school wrestlers, Weissinger et al. (1991) found current or past prevalences of the following pathogenic weight control behaviors in the sample: fasting, 51%; diet pills, 14%; diuretics, 10%; laxatives, 8%; and vomiting, 15%. Similarly, Steen and Brownell (1990) studied 63 college and 368 high school wrestlers and found that fasting was common among both college (63%) and high school athletes (44%), while vomiting and laxative and diuretic use were used by a smaller but significant percentage of athletes (2%-5%).

Jockeys represent another group of male athletes that are considered at high risk for disordered eating. Interestingly, despite the plethora of anecdotal reports describing bizarre dieting rituals and eating behaviors, there is surprisingly little scientific evidence of clinical eating disorders among jockeys. In fact, a search of the literature turned up only two studies examining eating disorders in jockeys conducted nearly 15 years apart. In the more recent of the two studies, (Leydon and Wall 2002) 20 jockeys (14 female and 6 male) were screened for disordered eating using the EAT-26 and a questionnaire developed by the authors that assessed methods for "making weight." Overall 20% of the jockeys (3 female and 1 male) had elevated EAT-26 scores (indicative of disordered eating) and 67% of the jockeys regularly engaged in one or more pathogenic weight loss method (e.g., severe food restriction, fasting, excessive exercise and the abuse of saunas, laxatives, and diuretics) in order to "make weight." Using similar instruments (i.e., the EAT-26 and a questionnaire assessing pathogenic weight loss methods) along with a follow-up clinical interview, King and Mezey (1987) examined disordered eating behaviors among 14 male jockeys. Although pathogenic weight control behaviors were commonly reported among the jockeys (ranging from 21% for fasting to 100% for excessive exercise), the authors concluded that, based on clinical evaluation, "no case of an eating disorder was found among the subjects" (King and Mezey 1987, p. 251). Moreover, while the majority of jockeys reported pathogenic weight control behaviors during the season, none reported continuation of these behaviors in the off-season.

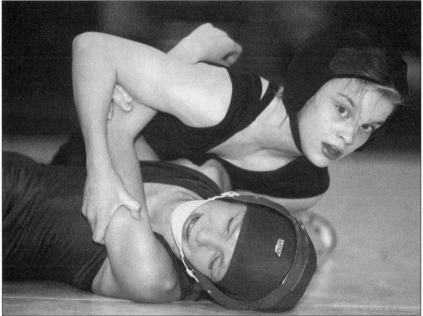

© Jim West

Contributing to the higher prevalence of disordered eating in female athletes is the fact that females are more likely to deem weight critical to performance. Female athletes also often report difficulty in attaining and maintaining both their own ideal competitive weight and the weight suggested by their coaches.

The transient disordered eating behaviors seen in these jockeys have also been reported in wrestlers (Dale and Landers 1999) and have led some researchers to question whether they are truly comparable to the behaviors of clinical eating disorder patients, whose obsession with dieting and weight loss persists endlessly (Mickalide 1990). Indeed, several researchers have argued that such "functional" dieting and subsequent weight loss differ markedly from a clinical eating disorder because they are a means to the end of athletic success (rather than an end in themselves) and generally the central pathology characteristic of clinical eating disorders is absent (Mickalide 1990).

Nonetheless, regardless of the authenticity of disordered eating in male athletes, the pathogenic weight control behaviors practiced by those with disordered eating can have devastating consequences on both health and performance. Moreover, researchers and practitioners agree that severe or chronic dieting can eventually develop into a full-blown eating disorder (Andersen 1992; Sundgot-Borgen et al. 1999). Indeed, both male and female athletes frequently report that their eating disorder was preceded by a period of dieting or stringent weight control (Sundgot-Borgen et al. 1999). In the study by Sundgot-Borgen and colleagues, dieting was one of the most commonly reported predisposing factors by both male (13%) and female (60%) athletes with eating disorders. Interestingly, the other commonly reported eating disorder risk factor for both male (25%) and female (28%) athletes was sustaining an injury.

Physiological and Health Consequences of Disordered Eating

The physiological responses to starvation or bingeing and purging are similar between males and females with disordered eating, and the similarities become more pronounced as the severity of the disorder increases (Andersen 1992; Andersen and Holman 1997). For example, both male and female anorexics often manifest bradycardia, hypotension, muscle wasting, cold intolerance, and endocrine abnormalities (decreased levels of sex hormones and decreased libido). Similarly, both males and females with bulimia nervosa suffer gastrointestinal distress, electrolyte imbalances, dental caries, generalized weakness, and potential kidney damage (Andersen 1992). (More on the health consequences of disordered eating is presented in chapter 6).

Differences

Despite some striking similarities there are distinct differences between males and females with disordered eating. Those differences include the developmental history, reasons for dieting, and pathogenic weight control methods used and are described below.

Developmental History of Disordered Eating

According to Andersen (1992), males who develop disordered eating are more likely to have actually been overweight or even obese (particularly those who develop bulimia nervosa), as opposed to females who simply felt overweight or obese. Thus, for the male with disordered eating, the fear of gaining weight or becoming fat is not completely irrational but rather is born out of past experience. This difference is supported by series of clinical case histories of male and female eating disorder patients reported by Andersen and Holman (1997). According to these studies, the average body mass index (BMI) for males (27.20 kg/m²) who went on to develop eating disorders fell into the range of objective medical obesity, while the average maximum BMI for females (24.34 kg/m²) was within the normal range.

Andersen (1992) also contends that males (both athletes and nonathletes) with disordered eating are less concerned with body weight (i.e., the number on the scale) than their female counterparts but are more concerned with body composition (i.e., percentage of lean body mass relative to fat mass). In addition, while both males and females with disordered eating suffer a similar degree of body dissatisfaction, females display a significantly greater desire for thinness. For example, Woodside and colleagues (1990) found that males with eating disorders scored significantly lower on the drive for

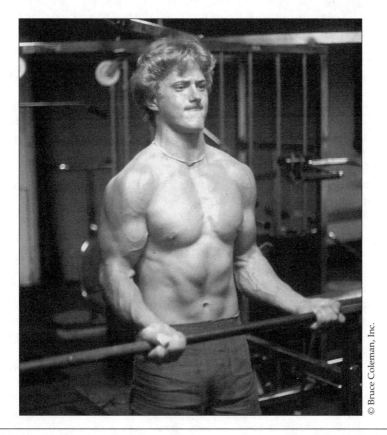

© Bruce Coleman, Inc.

Females with eating disorders universally want to lose weight. Males with eating disorders equally want to lose weight and gain weight through muscle mass.

thinness subscale of the EDI than females (11.57 vs. 17.15, respectively). A dichotomy in the direction of desired weight change is frequently found in males with eating disorders that is not seen in females. That is, females with disordered eating universally want to lose weight, while males tend to be evenly split between those wanting to lose weight and those desiring weight gain (Drenowski and Yee 1987). For example, Blouin and Goldfield (1995) found that male weightlifters presenting with significant body dissatisfaction displayed both a "drive for bulk" and a "drive for thinness." The authors attributed the apparently contradictory drives to the weightlifters' desire to increase lean body mass while decreasing body fat.

The sexual sphere is particularly salient in differentiating males and females with eating disorders. Research indicates that males with disordered eating more frequently report a history of conflict over gender identity or sexual orientation, whereas females tend more often to report a history of sexual abuse (Andersen 1992; Herzog, Bradburn, and Newman 1990). Crisp (1983) observed that uncertainty over gender identity was frequently present at the onset of anorexia nervosa in males, and several authors have reported that homosexual conflict preceded the onset of eating disorders in as many as 50% of male patients (Crisp 1967; Crisp and Toms 1972; Dally 1969; Herzog et al. 1984; Robinson and Holden 1986). Schneider and Agras (1987) matched male and female bulimics by age, duration of illness, and frequency of self-induced vomiting and found that 53% of the men but none of the women were homosexual or bisexual.

Although sexual histories or experiences may differ between males and females with eating disorders, the underlying motivation and resulting behaviors may be similar. That is, some researchers speculate that conflict over homosexual feelings in males with eating disorders plays a role comparable to that of heterosexual conflict in females with eating disorders. Reducing or eliminating sexual drive through starvation or bingeing and purging allows both males and females with eating disorders to resolve, at least temporarily, their sexual conflict (Andersen 1992).

Reasons for Dieting

As previously described, disordered eating in both males and females typically develops after a period of dieting that becomes increasingly stringent (anorexia nervosa) or increasingly erratic (bulimia nervosa). However, according to Andersen (1992), the factors *initiating* the dieting behavior may be different for males and females. In general, males with eating disorders diet as a means to an end, while for females, dieting is the end itself. For example, as described earlier, males who develop disordered eating are more likely to have actually had a history of overweight or obesity. They also more often report having been relentlessly teased or criticized for their weight. The psychological and emotional distress suffered as a result of the teasing is thought to instill a strong resolution to maintain a low body weight (e.g., a boy may vow never to be teased about his weight again; Andersen 1992).

Males are also more apt to begin dieting to avoid weight-related ill-nesses, particularly if they have witnessed such an illness in a family member (e.g., an overweight father with diabetes or heart disease; Andersen 1992). Finally, males more frequently report dieting to improve athleticism or enhance sport performance than do females. In a study reported by Andersen and Holman (1997), 44% of males diagnosed with eating disorders began dieting for one of these reasons (i.e., to prevent the recurrence of obesity and the teasing that resulted from it, to avoid weight-related medical complications, or to improve sport performance), whereas just 7% of females with eating disorders reported dieting for one or more of those reasons.

This last distinction between males and females with eating disor-ders—dieting to improve sport performance—is of particular relevance to athletes. Indeed, research suggests that male athletes more often diet to improve performance, whereas their female counterparts diet to enhance appearance (Andersen 1992; Fogelholm and Hilloskorpi 1999; Sundgot-Borgen 1994; Thompson and Sherman 1993). The reported sex differences in eating disorder incidence seem to support this notion, as the prevalence of eating disorders among female athletes tends to be highest in aesthetic sports (e.g., dance, gymnastics, and figure skating), whereas prevalence estimates are highest for males in endurance sports (e.g., cross-country running) and sports with weight classifications (e.g., wrestling; Sundgot-Borgen 1999). It has also been reported that male athletes are more likely than their female counterparts to engage in "defensive dieting," that is, dieting to prevent weight gain during an injury or illness (Thompson and Sherman 1993).

Methods of Dieting

According to Andersen (1992), males are more apt to use excessive exercise as a means of weight control, whereas females typically use more passive methods, such as severe energy restriction, vomiting, and laxative abuse. These weight control differences may stem from the societal biases sur-rounding dieting and male behavior; that is, dieting is considered to be more acceptable for women because the overwhelming sociocultural belief is that "real men don't diet." While excessive exercise may be viewed by some as less problematic than other pathogenic weight loss methods (e.g., vomiting and laxative abuse), there are some distinct disadvantages that are particularly relevant to the athlete. Excessive exercise invariably leads to *overtraining syndrome*, which is characterized by a marked decrease in performance and an increased risk for injury, both of which can serve to accelerate the progression or increase the severity of the eating disorder. Moreover, the obsession with exercise and fitness can lead to the indis-criminant use of nutritional supplements, including those that have been shown to be particularly dangerous (e.g., ephedrine and its alkaloids, anabolic steroids, and growth hormone; Mickalide 1990; Pope, Phillips, and Olivardia 2000).

Muscle Dysmorphia:
The "New" Male Eating Disorder?

A group of researchers have recently described a form of body image disturbance in male bodybuilders and weightlifters that they refer to as *muscle dysmorphia*. According to these researchers, muscle dysmorphia is a subtype of *body dysmorphic disorder,* which has been defined as an intense and excessive preoccupation or dissatisfaction with a perceived defect in appearance (see table 4.1). Once referred to as "reverse anorexia" (Pope and Katz 1994; Pope, Katz, and Hudson 1993), muscle dysmorphia is characterized by an inordinate preoccupation and dissatisfaction with body size and muscularity. Individuals with muscle dysmorphia perceive themselves as small and frail even though they are actually quite large and muscular.

Muscle dysmorphia shares some similarities with eating disorders: body image disturbance or distortion, preoccupation with body weight and size, excessive exercise, preoccupation with food and dieting, and use of pathogenic weight control behaviors. However, there are also some distinct differences (Pope et al. 1997). Individuals with muscle dysmorphia seek to increase body weight and size, whereas those with eating disorders are most often looking to decrease body weight or size. In addition, those with muscle dysmorphia frequently abuse performance-enhancing drugs and dietary supplements, particularly those that promise weight gain or muscle development (Pope and Katz 1994). In their initial report, Pope, Katz, and Hudson (1993) noted that 13% of weightlifters with muscle dysmorphia also reported a history of disordered eating and all reported a history of anabolic steroid abuse. In a more recent study (Pope, Phillips, and Olivardia 2000), one third of the weightlifters with muscle dysmorphia reported comorbid eating disorders, and more than half reported using anabolic steroids.

Although there are currently no universally accepted diagnostic criteria for muscle dysmorphia, a recent study by Olivardia, Pope, and Hudson (2000) offers some insight into possible distinguishing features. In this study male weightlifters from 23 Boston-area gymnasiums were screened for symptoms of muscle dysmorphia. The screening identified 23 weightlifters with pronounced muscle dysmorphia and 30 with no apparent body image distortions (control weightlifters). Using a variety of psychological questionnaires, the authors were able to identify some distinguishing features of those with muscle dysmorphia. Although physically the weightlifters with muscle dysmorphia resembled the control weightlifters (i.e., similar body weights and body fat percentages), those with muscle dysmorphia reported significantly more body image dissatisfaction, distortion, and preoccupation. The weightlifters with muscle dysmorphia expressed a significantly greater degree of body weight and shape dissatisfaction, more frequently reported "feeling fat," engaged in significantly more body weight and appearance appraisals (e.g., weighing themselves, checking themselves in mirrors or windows, seeking approval from friends and relatives about their body size and shape), and expressed a greater discomfort with the idea of

Table 4.1 Clinical Features and Diagnostic Criteria for Body Dysmorphic Disorder and Muscle Dysmorphia

Disorder	Clinical features and diagnostic criteria
Body dysmorphic disorder	• Preoccupation with a perceived physical defect. • Clinically significant distress or impairment in school, work, or social situations. • Preoccupation is not better explained by another mental disorder, such as anorexia nervosa.
Muscle dysmorphia	• The individual demonstrates a preoccupation with the idea of being not sufficiently lean and muscular. Behaviors associated with this preoccupation include frequent weighing; constant checking of appearance in mirrors or windows; persistent criticism of body weight, size, or shape; wearing baggy clothing to camouflage the body or, conversely, modifying clothing to accentuate muscularity (such as adding extra buttons to make shirt sleeves look tighter). • The preoccupation with muscularity causes clinically significant distress or impairment of social, occupational, or other important areas of life functioning (e.g., personal relationships) as demonstrated by at least two of the following: —The individual frequently gives up important social, occupational, or recreational activities because of a compulsive need to maintain an exercise and dietary regimen. —The individual avoids situations where his body would be exposed to others (e.g., at the beach or swimming pool) or endures such situations only with marked distress or intense anxiety. —The preoccupation about the inadequacy of body size or muscularity causes clinically significant distress or impairment in social, occupational, or other important areas of life. —The individual continues to exercise, diet, or use performance-enhancing drugs or supplements, despite knowledge of adverse physical or psychological consequences. • The individual engages in excessive exercise, demonstrates preoccupation with food, follows strict dietary regimens (e.g., avoiding specific foods or groups of foods, maintaining an excessively low-fat or high-protein diet), or abuses steroids or dietary supplements, particularly those aimed at increasing body size (e.g., creatine, HMB [beta-hydroxy-beta-methylbutyrate], DHEA [dihydroepiandrosterone], androstenedione) or decreasing body fat (e.g., ephedrine, ma huang, guarana).

having to expose their bodies (e.g., taking their shirt off at a beach) than the control weightlifters. In addition, those with muscle dysmorphia reported higher rates of current or past major mood, anxiety, or eating disorders than the control weightlifters (Olivardia, Pope, and Hudson 2000).

Summary

Anecdotal evidence and the limited existing research suggest that females with eating disorders greatly outnumber males. The limited available data indicate that the dichotomy in eating disorder prevalence likely holds true for athletes as well.

The reasons for this eating disorder gender gap are numerous and complex. Researchers most often cite the disparity in sociocultural and sport-specific expectations regarding body weight as well as biological, hormonal, and evolutionary differences between the sexes for the higher eating disorder prevalence in females than in males. Differences in prevalence aside, most researchers and clinicians agree that males and females with disordered eating are probably more similar than dissimilar and that the similarities tend to become greater with increasing severity of the disorder. Nonetheless, some important differences do exist. Males suffering from disordered eating are distinctive in their increased probability of having a history of overweight or obesity, their more common use of defensive dieting to avoid medical illness or weight gain as a result of an injury, and the equal likelihood of their desiring weight loss or weight gain. Moreover, the newly identified body image disorder, muscle dysmorphia, is almost exclusively found in males, particularly male bodybuilders and weightlifters.

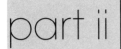

part ii

Effects of Disordered Eating

five

Effects of Disordered Eating on Performance

CHAPTER OBJECTIVES

After reading this chapter, you will be able to

- describe the effects of chronic or restrictive dieting on athletic performance and

- describe the effects of bingeing and purging on athletic performance.

Muscular work requires energy, namely, calories. Failure to provide the muscles with adequate energy, particularly in the form of carbohydrates, is like forgetting to fill up your gas tank before a long road trip; you will inevitably run out of gas before reaching your destination. Athletes who chronically restrict calories or binge and purge are basically "running on empty." Thus, they are likely to suffer premature fatigue and poor performance.

This chapter focuses on the effects of disordered eating on athletic performance. Because there is limited data detailing the direct cause-and-effect consequences of disordered eating on athletic performance, much of the information provided is more indirect or theoretical in nature.

Effects of Chronic or Restrictive Dieting on Performance

It seems logical to assume that chronic energy restriction and the resulting inadequate macronutrient (i.e., carbohydrate, protein, and fat) and micronutrient (i.e., vitamins and minerals) intakes cause a decrement in athletic performance. Nonetheless, to date there is little *direct* evidence supporting this contention, largely because it is difficult to accurately measure energy or nutrient intakes in athletes over an extended period. Moreover, it is difficult to make causal associations between long-term nutrient inadequacies and performance because of the difficulty in controlling possible confounding factors.

Surprisingly, anecdotal evidence (i.e., reports from coaches and personal accounts by athletes with disordered eating) suggests that severe energy restriction and the resulting weight loss are actually associated with an initial, albeit transient, *increase* in performance. The reasons for this temporary increase in performance are not completely understood but may be related to the initial physiological and psychological consequences of starvation (Johnson 1994). As a physiological stressor, starvation produces an up-regulation of the hypothalamic-pituitary-adrenal axis, better known as the fight-or-flight response. The result is an increase in the adrenal hormones—cortisol, epinephrine, and norepinephrine—which have stimulatory effects on the central nervous system. High circulating levels of these hormones may produce a high-energy state and evoke a sense of excitability and exhilaration in the energy-restricting athlete.

In addition, the initial decrease in body weight (particularly before there is a significant decrease in muscle mass) may induce a transient increase in *relative* $\dot{V}O_2$max (maximal oxygen uptake per kilogram of body weight). Since $\dot{V}O_2$max reflects the body's capacity to perform aerobic or endurance exercise, an increase may translate into an improvement in endurance performance, at least over the short term (Fogelholm 1994; Ingjer and Sundgot-Borgen 1991). Moreover, with weight loss, athletes may *feel* lighter, which may afford them a psychological boost, particularly if they subscribe to the belief that lighter always means faster; however, no data indicate that lighter runners, swimmers, divers, gymnasts, or other athletes are faster or perform better. Finally, we cannot discount the possibility that the initial increase in performance is drug induced. Athletes seeking quick weight loss often resort to using diet pills or ingesting large quantities of caffeine or other stimulants to decrease appetite and maintain energy levels in the face of inadequate energy intake. The stimulatory effects of these drugs may be strong enough to override the effects of malnutrition and the resulting fatigue, especially in the early stages of severe energy restriction. It should be emphasized, however, that the increase in performance sometimes seen with energy restriction is only *temporary*. Eventually, the body will break down and performance will suffer (see the sidebar; Beals and Manore 1994).

The effects of energy restriction on athletic performance are a function of the severity and chronicity of the energy restriction and of the physiological demands of the sport. Thus, an individual who engages in severe energy restriction or who has been restricting energy for a long time will likely experience a greater decrement in performance than one who has engaged in milder energy restriction for a shorter time. Likewise, energy restriction is apt to have different effects depending on the type and intensity of the exercise performed. That is, endurance sports and other physical activities with high energy demands (e.g., distance running, swimming, cycling, basketball, field and ice hockey) are likely to be more negatively affected by energy restriction than sports with lower energy demands (e.g., diving, gymnastics, weightlifting). Similarly, athletes who train at a high intensity (e.g., elite athletes) are apt to suffer greater performance decrements with energy restriction than those who engage in lower-intensity exercise (e.g., recreational athletes).

Physiological Effects of Severe or Rapid Weight Loss

Severe or rapid weight loss, particularly if it is achieved via pathogenic methods, can be detrimental to athletic performance. These are some of the physiological effects of severe or rapid weight loss and their potential impact on performance:

Physiological effect	Effect on performance
Glycogen depletion	• Premature muscular fatigue (muscle glycogen depletion) • Reduced mental capacity or psychological fatigue (liver glycogen depletion)
Increased lactate production	• Impaired buffering capacity • Premature muscular fatigue

(continued)

Physiological effect	Effect on performance
Dehydration	• Impaired thermoregulation (increased risk of heat cramps, heat exhaustion, and heatstroke) • Impaired oxygen transport and nutrient exchange • Premature muscular fatigue
Loss of lean body mass	• Reduced muscular strength and endurance • Decreased anaerobic performance
Reduced cardiac output	• Decreased aerobic (endurance) capacity

The decrement in performance seen with chronic or severe energy restriction is likely due to one or more of the following factors:

- Nutrient deficiencies
- Fatigue
- Frequent infection and illness
- Iron deficiency
- Frequent injuries
- Reduced cardiovascular function

Nutrient Deficiencies

Chronic or severe energy restriction is directly associated with inadequate nutrient intakes that eventually lead to nutrient deficiencies and a decrement in athletic performance. Indeed, it is nearly impossible for an active individual consuming fewer than 1,200 kcal/d to meet macronutrient (i.e., carbohydrate, protein, and fat) and micronutrient (i.e., vitamin and mineral) requirements. Athletes suffering from disordered eating often avoid carbohydrate-rich foods (e.g., bread, pasta, rice, cereals) for fear that these foods will promote weight gain or inhibit weight loss. This is unfortunate, because inadequate carbohydrate intake (<5 g/kg in women and <7 g/kg in men; Coyle 1995) compromises both muscle and liver glycogen stores. The result is a more rapid onset of muscular weakness (muscle glycogen depletion) and mental fatigue (liver glycogen depletion and subsequent low blood glucose) during exercise. Studies have consistently shown that carbohydrate restriction negatively affects athletic performance, particularly endurance performance (Coogan and Coyle 1987; Coyle 1995; O'Keefe et al. 1989; Simonsen et al. 1991).

An athlete consuming insufficient calories is also likely not getting enough protein to synthesize and maintain lean body mass and to replace any protein used for energy during exercise. While protein typically contributes 15% or less of the fuel used during exercise, the amount may be considerably larger if carbohydrate (i.e., glucose) is in short supply or if energy intake is low (i.e., during periods of dieting; Lemon 1995). Without enough protein to maintain and repair muscle tissue, the athlete increases his or her risk of muscle wasting, weakness, and injury.

Fat restriction or even elimination often goes hand in hand with energy restriction. If fat intake is too low (<10% of total energy intake), the intake and absorption of fat-soluble vitamins and essential fatty acids are likely also to be low, which can lead to fatigue and poor athletic performance (Manore and Thompson 2000).

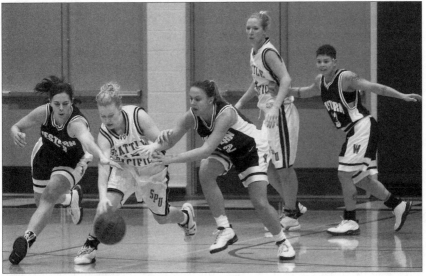

© Dale Garvey

Athletes in endurance sports with high energy demands, such as distance running and basketball, are more likely to be negatively affected by energy restriction than athletes in sports with lower energy demands.

Finally, athletes with inadequate energy intake are also likely to have poor vitamin and mineral intakes. This is particularly true for the B-complex vitamins (thiamin, riboflavin, niacin, vitamin B_6, folate, and vitamin B_{12}) and the minerals iron, calcium, zinc, and magnesium (Manore 1996, 1998). These micronutrients are especially important for the athlete because they play central roles in energy production, hemoglobin synthesis, muscle tissue synthesis and repair, bone health, and immune function (Manore and Thompson 2000). Poor micronutrient status thus can lead to fatigue, muscle weakness, musculoskeletal injuries, and an increased risk of infections (Manore 1996, 1998).

Fatigue

Constant or severe energy restriction and the subsequent rapid weight loss that often accompanies it can contribute to a state of chronic fatigue in the athlete (Eichner 1992). The fatigue may be experienced only when the athlete exercises, or it may be a more generalized, constant fatigue that is experienced during nontraining times as well.

As discussed earlier, inadequate energy intake is typically associated with inadequate carbohydrate consumption. Failure to replenish muscle glycogen stores leads to muscle glycogen depletion, which is a primary factor contributing to fatigue in athletes during training and competition. Moreover, liver glycogen depletion can lead to a chronic state of low blood glucose, which is associated with a feeling of generalized fatigue (Coyle 1995).

Finally, if energy intake is inadequate, it is highly likely that iron intake is inadequate as well. Suboptimal iron intake can lead to iron-deficiency anemia, a condition characterized by both generalized and local muscular fatigue that typically worsens with exercise (Nielson and Nachtigall 1998). Iron deficiency is discussed in more detail later in this chapter.

Frequent Infection and Illness

Common sense suggests that malnutrition resulting from chronic or severe energy restriction places an athlete at increased risk of infection. Nonetheless, to date there is little direct evidence that disordered eating, at least in the early stages, predisposes the athlete to developing infections or illnesses (Eichner 1992). In fact, research suggests that the risk of infection does not increase significantly in individuals with anorexia or bulimia nervosa until the advanced stages of the disorders. For example, an early study examining the effect of anorexia nervosa on infection risk found that the incidence of infection in anorexic patients was not clearly increased above normal despite substantially lower total leukocyte counts and lower absolute neutrophil, lymphocyte, and monocyte counts (Bowers and Eckert 1978). Similarly, the decreases in immunoglobulin levels and impaired cellular immunity often seen with anorexia nervosa are modest until the individual reaches the point of extreme malnutrition (Eichner 1992).

Thus, it remains unclear whether the typical athlete with disordered eating is at increased risk for illness or infection. Nonetheless, it seems reasonable to assume that chronic or severe energy restriction combined with the high energy expenditure characteristic of most athletes with disordered eating can lead to increasing malnutrition that eventually compromises the immune system and increases the risk of infection.

Iron Deficiency

It is nearly impossible to obtain adequate dietary iron if energy intake is low. Thus, it is no surprise that chronic or severe energy restriction frequently leads to iron deficiency. Indeed, iron-deficiency anemia is said to occur in

30% of patients with anorexia nervosa (Eichner 1992). Athletes, particularly endurance athletes, are also known to be at increased risk for poor iron status because of inadequate iron intake combined with increased iron loss (Weaver and Rajaram 1992). High-impact exercise (e.g., running and jumping) and exercise that creates high mechanical stress (e.g., weightlifting) can destroy red blood cells (i.e., hemolysis) and muscle cells, thereby releasing hemoglobin and myoglobin into the bloodstream, which are then excreted by the kidneys (hematuria). In addition, losses of iron in the sweat can be significant, particularly if the athlete is exercising in a hot or humid environment (Waller and Haymes 1996). Failure to compensate for these increased iron losses results in an iron deficiency. Thus, the athlete with disordered eating, who is likely consuming inadequate amounts of iron while experiencing significant losses, is at an exceptionally high risk for iron deficiency.

Without question, iron-deficiency anemia (i.e., below-normal hemoglobin levels) negatively affects performance. Hemoglobin is required for the transportation and utilization of oxygen and the clearance of carbon dioxide. In a hemoglobin-deficient state, the body is unable to supply adequate oxygen to and clear carbon dioxide from the working muscles. Inadequate oxygen supply to the muscle significantly decreases muscle function. Moreover, without adequate oxygen the muscles cannot oxidize fat; thus, there is increased reliance on carbohydrate, which can lead to more rapid glycogen depletion and lactic acid production. All of this results in a significant decrease in aerobic performance (and perhaps anaerobic performance as well).

Whether iron deficiency without anemia (i.e., either iron depletion or iron-deficiency erythropoiesis) compromises physiological function in the same manner or to the same extent as iron-deficiency anemia remains controversial (see table 5.1). However, consensus seems to hold that both iron depletion and iron deficiency erythropoiesis without anemia can negatively affect athletic performance, particularly endurance performance, albeit not to the same extent as iron-deficiency anemia (Hinton et al. 2000; Lukaski, Hall, and Siders 1991; Newhouse and Clement 1995). Moreover, because successful treatment of iron-deficiency anemia is such a difficult and lengthy process (i.e., it often takes more than four to six months for hemoglobin levels to return to normal), it is prudent to identify and treat iron deficiency in the early stages, before iron-deficiency anemia develops and performance is severely impaired.

Frequent Injuries

It is generally accepted that failure to provide the body with adequate energy and the nutrients necessary to build and repair tissue damaged by strenuous exercise increases the incidence of musculoskeletal injuries (Beals and Manore 1994). Inadequate energy leaves the body deficient of the carbohydrates and fats needed to fuel muscular work. Similarly, without adequate protein and micronutrients—zinc, calcium, magnesium, and vitamins C, E, and B_6, to name a few—tissue damaged by strenuous exercise cannot be repaired. Despite this obvious negative consequence of severe or chronic energy

Table 5.1 Stages of Iron Deficiency

Stage of deficiency	Physiological effects	Clinical manifestation	Effect on performance
Iron depletion (prelatent)	• Iron stores (ferritin) are significantly lowered.	Plasma ferritin ≤ 12 μg/L	Questionable. Iron-dependent enzymes involved in fat metabolism may be inhibited, causing increases in glucose oxidation and lactic acid production and premature fatigue due to glycogen depletion (particularly during endurance exercise).
Iron-deficiency erythropoiesis (latent)	• Iron levels in the blood are reduced. • Ability to synthesize new red blood cells is decreased.	• Plasma ferritin ≤ 12 μg/L • Total iron-binding capacity (TIBC) > 4,000 μg/L • Transferrin saturation < 16% • Plasma iron < 500 μg/L	Questionable. Reduced iron availability and decreased red blood cell formation could compromise oxygen delivery to muscle cells, thereby impairing athletic performance (particularly endurance performance).
Iron-deficiency anemia	• Red blood cell number and size are decreased. • Oxygen transport to and carbon dioxide clearance from body tissues is compromised.	• Plasma ferritin ≤ 12 μg/L • TIBC > 4,000 μg/L • Transferrin saturation < 16% • Plasma iron < 500 μg/L • Hemoglobin < 120 mg/L • Hematocrit < 36% • Hypochromic, microcytic red blood cells	Endurance performance is significantly decreased. Reduced hemoglobin levels result in decreased oxygen delivery to and carbon dioxide clearance from body tissues. Without adequate oxygen, fat oxidation is reduced and reliance on glucose for fuel increases, causing lactic acid accumulation and more rapid glycogen depletion.

Adapted, by permission, from M.M. Manore and J. Thompson, 2000, *Sport nutrition for health & performance* (Champaign, IL: Human Kinetics), 345.

restriction, few studies have directly assessed the impact of energy restriction on injury rates in athletes. Nonetheless, indirect evidence and anecdotal reports suggest a higher rate of injuries among athletes who restrict energy intake or practice disordered eating behaviors. For example, research indicates that athletes in thin-build sports (where the pressure to be thin is high and dieting is common) report poor energy and nutrient intakes, are at increased risk of injury, and report a prolonged recovery time from injury (Beals and Manore 2002; Beckvid-Henriksson, Schnell, and Linden-Hirschberg 2000). For example, a recent study by Beals and Manore (2002) found that collegiate athletes in thin-build sports reported more musculoskeletal injuries than those in sports that do not emphasize a thin build. In addition, athletes suffering from disordered eating sustained more bone injuries during their collegiate athletic careers than those who did not report disordered eating.

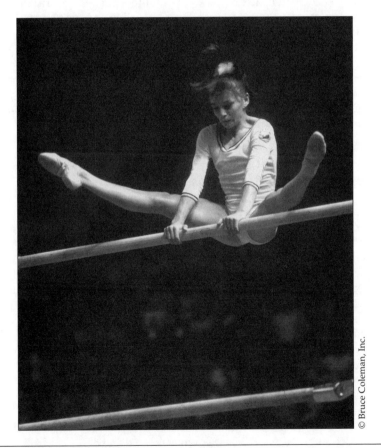

© Bruce Coleman, Inc.

Research indicates that athletes in thin-build sports, where dieting is common (such as gymnastics), report poor energy and nutrient intakes and a prolonged recovery time from injury.

Reduced Cardiovascular Function

The cardiovascular changes associated with anorexia nervosa (e.g., bradycardia, generalized and orthostatic hypotension, reductions in cardiac chamber size and wall thickness, and electrocardiographic abnormalities [Eichner 1992; Carney and Andersen 1996]) can have serious repercussions on athletic performance, particularly endurance performance or that which involves aerobic exercise. The extent to which performance will be impacted by these cardiovascular abnormalities depends on the severity and duration of the energy restriction and the physical demands of the athlete's training regimen. If the energy restriction causes a significant decrease in the size and strength of the heart muscle, cardiac function will be compromised and aerobic capacity reduced. Specifically, a decrease in cardiac musculature results in reduced stroke volume (i.e., the amount of blood pumped by the heart with each heart beat, expressed in milliliters per beat) and a subsequent reduction in cardiac output (i.e., the amount of blood pumped by the heart per minute), thereby reducing maximal exercise capacity.

A study by Ingjer and Sundgot-Borgen (1991) supports the negative consequences of severe restriction on cardiovascular function and athletic performance. These researchers found a significant decrease in maximal oxygen uptake and running speed of elite, endurance-trained female athletes both during and for several months after an intense two-month weight-reduction period.

Effects of Purging on Performance

As previously described, individuals with bulimia nervosa may purge by using one or more of several techniques, including use of diuretics, laxatives, or enemas; self-induced vomiting; or exercising excessively to burn off calories. If the purging methods place the athlete in a state of negative energy balance, then the potential effects on performance are similar to those seen with chronic or severe energy restriction, namely, nutrient deficiencies, fatigue, frequent injuries, cardiovascular abnormalities, and increased risk of infections or illnesses (see the sidebar). In addition, the gastrointestinal blood losses that often result from chronic vomiting can contribute to iron losses and increase the risk of iron-deficiency anemia. Excessive exercise, especially given inadequate energy and nutrient intakes, invariably leads to overuse injuries. In addition to the resulting energy and nutrient deficiencies, purging poses some unique problems regarding athletic performance, most notably dehydration and electrolyte abnormalities.

Is Purging an Effective Method of Weight Control?

Many athletes believe that purging will promote rapid and effective weight loss and prevent weight gain associated with frequent bingeing. In fact, most purging methods not only are ineffective in promoting weight loss (and preventing weight gain) but can have severe consequences on the health and performance of the athlete.

Self-Induced Vomiting and Laxative and Diuretic Use

Self-induced vomiting may only remove one third to one half of what has been eaten. Digestion and absorption of food is a very rapid and efficient process. Most of the food consumed at a given meal empties from the stomach within 15 to 20 minutes after consumption, and absorption occurs within minutes thereafter. Even vomiting immediately after eating does not prevent the body from absorbing some calories. Thus, the weight loss associated with self-induced vomiting is minimal and can be attributed primarily to the loss of body fluids that accompanies vomiting.

Similarly, laxatives and diuretics induce the loss of primarily water (along with important minerals, including electrolytes), not consumed food. Laxatives cause an increase in gastric motility (movement), but mainly through the colon, not the small intestine. Thus, the effect on nutrient absorption in the small intestine is minimal; however, the effect on the absorption of water and electrolytes in the colon is significant, such that considerable amounts of both are lost in the feces. Diuretics stimulate the formation and excretion of urine by the kidneys. Thus, the minimal weight that is lost via these purging methods is body water, not body fat, which can result in dangerous dehydration and electrolyte imbalances.

In fact, not only are these purging techniques relatively ineffective for weight loss, but repetitive purging can, paradoxically, cause weight gain due to rebound water retention. When the body becomes dehydrated, a variety of hormones are secreted in an attempt to restore normal fluid balance. These hormones (aldosterone, angiotensin, and renin) act on the kidney, causing it to retain water and sodium. This increase in water retention, which is particularly noticeable in between purging episodes, may lead to a 2- to 5-lb (0.9- to 2.3-kg) weight gain in as little as 24 hours.

Excessive Exercise

Excessive exercise has only recently been recognized as a form of purging. With athletes in particular it may be difficult to determine what constitutes "excessive" exercise or physical training. Nonetheless, it is generally accepted that exercise should be considered excessive if it is over and above that required for normal training and is done solely for the purpose of burning extra calories. Exercise as a purging technique is effective only if the additional exercise creates a state of negative energy balance or can burn off the calories consumed during a binge. This is highly unlikely, however, as a binge can involve consuming as much as 5,000 kcal in one sitting. Numerous hours of exercise would be required to burn off that many calories.

More likely, excessive exercise as a purging technique will lead only to an overuse injury. The injury will then render the athlete unable to exercise, which can lead the athlete to use other forms of purging (e.g., self-induced vomiting, use of laxatives or diuretics) or severe energy restriction in an attempt to prevent weight gain.

Reprinted, by permission, from C.L. Otis and R. Goldingay, 2000, *The athletic woman's survival guide* (Champaign, IL: Human Kinetics), 96.

Dehydration

Diuretics, laxatives, and self-induced vomiting all cause a loss of body fluid, albeit via slightly different mechanisms. Diuretics stimulate the formation and excretion of urine by the kidney. Laxatives increase gastric motility through the colon, thereby decreasing the amount of fluid and electrolytes reabsorbed and increasing the amount lost in the feces. The fluid lost with self-induced vomiting is largely from gastrointestinal juices.

Dehydration is one of the most common nutritional causes of premature fatigue and poor athletic performance (Manore and Thompson 2000). A loss of just 1% of body weight as water can negatively affect performance (Greenleaf 1992; Manore and Thompson 2000). Dehydration hastens the onset of fatigue and raises the perceived exertion (i.e., the exercise feels harder than it would in a well-hydrated state; Maughan 1992; Manore and Thompson 2000). In addition, when a person exercises while dehydrated, glycogen is used more rapidly; thus, glycogen depletion occurs sooner than it would in a well-hydrated state.

The most serious consequence of dehydration, however, is the reduction in plasma volume and the resulting decreased blood flow to the skin, which decreases the body's ability to cool itself via the evaporation of sweat and the radiation of heat. This in turn raises the body's core temperature and increases the risk of muscle cramps, heat exhaustion, and the more dangerous condition of heatstroke (Manore and Thompson 2000).

Self-induced vomiting and laxative and diuretic abuse can all promote dehydration. While these purging techniques are a health risk to anyone who practices them, they are particularly dangerous for the athlete, as they accelerate the water loss that occurs with exercise. That is, a purging athlete is likely to enter a training bout or competition already in a hypohydrated state; the exercise exacerbates water loss, and dehydration may ensue more quickly. The result is a more rapid onset of muscular and mental fatigue and a greater risk of heat illnesses.

Electrolyte Abnormalities

Self-induced vomiting and the abuse of laxatives and diuretics can lead to a loss of electrolytes, particularly potassium. Indeed, a low potassium level, also known as *hypokalemia,* is one of the clinical signs frequently used to identify bulimia nervosa. Physical symptoms associated with hypokalemia include generalized weakness, confusion, nausea, heart palpitations, abdominal pain, and constipation. In addition, low potassium levels can raise the risk of cardiac arrhythmia. From a performance standpoint, hypokalemia can cause local muscular fatigue and increase the risk of muscle cramps, particularly if the individual is suffering from dehydration as well (Eichner 1992).

Summary

Despite the lack of direct scientific evidence, the limited indirect evidence as well as common sense suggest that disordered eating behaviors impair athletic performance. Chronic or severe energy restriction and purging deprive the body of the energy necessary to fuel the muscles, the carbohydrate needed for glycogen replacement, the protein required for tissue synthesis and repair, and the micronutrients essential for energy metabolism and the maintenance of body homeostasis. Moreover, purging via self-induced vomiting or diuretic and laxative abuse poses the additional problems of dehydration and electrolyte imbalances.

Thus, the result of disordered eating behaviors is typically not an improvement in performance, as the athlete intends, but quite the opposite. An athlete who engages in chronic or severe energy restriction or purging is likely to suffer multiple nutritional deficiencies, chronic fatigue, and dehydration and is at an increased risk of dangerous electrolyte imbalances, none of which are conducive to optimal athletic performance.

six

Effects of Disordered Eating on Health

CHAPTER OBJECTIVES

After reading this chapter, you will be able to

- describe the effects of severe or chronic energy restriction on an athlete's health,

- identify the health risks associated with menstrual dysfunction in athletes (specifically the risk of low bone mineral density), and

- describe the effects of bingeing and purging on an athlete's health.

Chapter 5 described how the severe energy restriction and purging behaviors characteristic of individuals with disordered eating can negatively affect athletic performance. Of perhaps even greater concern are the potentially devastating effects that disordered eating behaviors can have on an athlete's health. While there is a vast amount of research documenting the medical complications of eating disorders in the general population, to date no studies have specifically examined the myriad health effects that disordered eating poses to athletes. Nonetheless, it can be assumed that the medical complications suffered by athletes with disordered eating are similar to those suffered by nonathletes with disordered eating (see table 6.1).

Table 6.1 Health Consequences of Various Pathogenic Weight Control Behaviors

Weight control behavior	Physiological effects and health consequences
Fasting or starvation	Promotes loss of lean body mass, a decrease in metabolic rate, and a reduction in bone mineral density. Increases the risk of nutrient deficiencies. Promotes glycogen depletion, resulting in poor exercise performance.
Diet pills	Typically function by suppressing appetite and may cause a slight increase in metabolic rate (if they contain ephedrine or caffeine). May induce rapid heart rate, anxiety, inability to concentrate, nervousness, inability to sleep, and dehydration. Any weight lost is quickly regained once use is discontinued.
Diuretics	Weight loss is primarily water, and any weight lost is quickly regained once use is discontinued. Dehydration and electrolyte imbalances are common and may disrupt thermoregulatory function and induce cardiac arrhythmia.
Laxatives or enemas	Weight loss is primarily water, and any weight lost is quickly regained once use is discontinued. Dehydration and electrolyte imbalances, constipation, cathartic colon (a condition in which the colon becomes unable to function properly on its own), and steatorrhea (excessive fat in the feces) are common. May be addictive, and athlete can develop resistance, thus requiring larger and larger doses to produce the same effect (or even to induce a normal bowel movement).
Self-induced vomiting	Largely ineffective in promoting weight (body fat) loss. Large body water losses can lead to dehydration and electrolyte imbalances. Gastrointestinal problems, including esophagitis, esophageal perforation, and esophageal and stomach ulcers, are common. May promote erosion of tooth enamel and increase the risk for dental caries. Finger calluses and abrasions are often present.

Weight control behavior	Physiological effects and health consequences
Fat-free diets	May be lacking in essential nutrients, especially fat-soluble vitamins and essential fatty acids. Total energy intake must still be reduced to produce weight loss. Many fat-free convenience foods are highly processed, with high sugar contents and few micronutrients unless the foods are fortified. The diet is often difficult to follow and may promote binge eating.
Saunas	Weight loss is primarily water, and any weight lost is quickly regained once fluids are replaced. Dehydration and electrolyte imbalances are common and may disrupt thermoregulatory function and induce cardiac arrhythmia.
Excessive exercise	Increases risk of staleness, chronic fatigue, illness, overuse injuries, and menstrual dysfunction.

Adapted, by permission, from C. Otis, 1998, "Too slim, amenorrheic, fracture-prone: The female-athlete triad," *ACSM's Health and Fitness Journal* 2(1): 20-25.

The morbidity associated with disordered eating can be explained by (1) the restriction of calories and the resulting state of starvation or semistarvation and (2) the purging techniques used to rid the body of ingested calories. This chapter describes the physiological and psychological consequences of disordered eating behaviors and the impact that these behaviors have on the overall health and well-being of the athlete.

Health Effects of Chronic and Severe Energy Restriction

As described in chapter 5, athletes who chronically or severely restrict energy intake likely suffer from macro- and micronutrient deficiencies, anemia, chronic fatigue, and an increased risk of infections and illnesses, all of which have the potential to harm both their performance and their health. Additional health effects associated with chronic or severe energy restriction and the resulting weight loss (or maintenance of a dangerously low body weight) include decreased basal metabolic rate, cardiovascular and gastrointestinal disorders, depression, menstrual dysfunction, and decreased bone mineral density.

Decreased Basal Metabolic Rate

Basal metabolic rate (BMR) is defined as the amount of energy expended at rest. It is estimated that BMR constitutes approximately 60% to 75% of total daily energy expenditure in a moderately active individual. In an elite or highly competitive athlete, it may account for somewhat less (about

50%-55%) because the amount of energy expended in physical activity is generally much higher. Despite these differences, for most individuals, including most athletes, BMR accounts for a significantly large (if not the largest) proportion of total daily energy expenditure.

Numerous studies have shown that energy restriction, particularly that of a severe or chronic nature, is associated with a decrease in BMR (Astrup et al. 1999; Brownell, Steen, and Wilmore 1987; Leibel, Rosenbaum, and Hirsch 1995; Thompson and Manore 1996; Weinsier, Hunter, and Schutz 2001; Weyer et al. 2000). Because of the significant contribution of BMR to total daily energy expenditure, a reduction in BMR results in a substantial reduction in the total amount of energy expended in a day. Fewer calories expended means that fewer calories are required to maintain body weight *and* that the degree of caloric restriction required for additional weight loss becomes even greater.

The decline in BMR seen with energy restriction is largely a result of the decrease in lean body mass that typically accompanies weight loss. However, some limited research indicates that the reduction in BMR that accompanies energy restriction is slightly greater than what would be predicted based on changes in lean body mass alone (Ravussin et al. 1982; Rosenbaum et al. 2000). This reduction in BMR, independent of lean body mass, is hypothesized to be caused by alterations in thyroid hormone function or activity. More specifically, it is believed that energy restriction causes an adaptive hypothyroidism resulting from an inhibition of the conversion of the relatively inactive thyroid hormone thyroxine (T4) to the more active triiodothyronine (T3; Brook and Marshal 1996).

Regardless of the precise physiological mechanism, experts agree that the decline in BMR is the body's protective response to energy restriction. That is, if the body is not receiving the energy it requires, then it will compensate by decreasing energy requirements. It also stands to reason, then, that whatever the body is defending might be further threatened by the additional energy demands of intense exercise. Thus, the reduction in BMR could be even greater in an athlete who is exercising strenuously *and* severely restricting energy intake. Logic also dictates that the reduction in BMR should be most pronounced in athletes who are attempting to achieve or maintain a weight that is significantly below their natural body weight (Brownell, Steen, and Wilmore 1997). Indeed, as the next section reveals, there is some evidence to suggest that the body in effect responds to a reduction in energy provisions by lowering its energy requirements.

Increased Energy and Food Efficiency

Some limited research suggests that severe or chronic energy restriction not only produces an adaptive decline in BMR but also may cause a decrease in the energy required to perform a given physical task (i.e., increased energy efficiency) as well as the number of calories required to maintain a given body weight or composition (i.e., increased food efficiency; Apfelbaum,

Bostsarron, and Lucatis 1971; Boyle, Storlien, and Keesey 1978; Brownell, Steen, and Wilmore 1987; Clark et al. 1992; Mulligan and Butterfield 1990; Thompson and Blanton 1987; Thompson, Manore, and Skinner 1993; Tuschl et al. 1990). For example, Tuschl et al. (1990) examined energy expenditure in a sample of young (18-30 yr), normal-weight (BMI 18-24 kg/m²) women classified as either restrained or unrestrained eaters. Despite the fact that the mean body weight of the restrained group was higher than that of the unrestrained group, both energy intake and energy expenditure were significantly lower (410 kcal/d and 620 kcal/d lower, respectively). Similarly, Apfelbaum, Bostsarron, and Lucatis (1971) found a 12% to 29% decrease in oxygen consumption in subjects performing a standard exercise task following diet restriction. It should be noted that not all studies support this energy conservation hypothesis (Schulz et al. 1992; Wilmore et al. 1992). However, these latter studies did not examine *dieting* athletes specifically, but rather amenorrheic and eumenorrheic (normally menstruating) female distance runners (with the assumption that the amenorrheic athletes were dieting).

If we assume that some degree of energy or food efficiency occurs in athletes who restrict energy intake, we can begin to understand the frustration that plagues them and how that frustration can lead to disordered eating. The following scenario illustrates this hypothetical sequence of events.

An athlete unhappy with his body weight restricts energy intake severely and subsequently loses weight. The weight loss leads to a decrease in energy expenditure and increased food efficiency. The energy and food efficiency then require the athlete to become ever more restrictive with energy intake. In effect, the athlete faces a never-ending food-restriction and body-weight battle. With increasing frustration over the plateaus in body weight, the athlete may begin to engage in more pathogenic dieting practices (e.g., self-induced vomiting, dehydration, and the use of diet pills and laxatives).

Cardiovascular Changes

The cardiovascular changes resulting from anorexia nervosa are well documented and include bradycardia, low blood pressure, and a decrease in heart chamber size and wall thickness (particularly of the left ventricle) that can result in mitral valve prolapse (i.e., prolapse of the mitral valve allowing blood from the left ventricle to seep back into the left atrium), and electrocardiographic abnormalities such as low voltage, T-wave inversion, and ST-segment depression (Eichner 1992; Carney and Andersen 1996). Whether the athlete who chronically restricts energy intake will suffer similar cardiovascular problems likely depends on the severity and chronicity of the energy restriction as well as the amount, rate, and composition of weight loss. If the liquid diet fiasco of the 1970s (in which 58 cardiac-related deaths were attributed to consumption of very low calorie, protein- and micronutrient-deficient liquid diets; Pomeroy and Mitchell 1992) is any indication, we might conclude that the potential deleterious effects on the athlete's cardiac function could be considerable.

Gastrointestinal Complications

Gastrointestinal (GI) complications associated with severe or chronic energy restriction result largely from the catabolic effects of starvation on the GI tract. Frequently, gastric motility is slowed, which results in delayed gastric empty-ing and contributes to abdominal bloating and feelings of fullness (Pomeroy and Mitchell 1992). Nonspecific abdominal pain and constipation are also commonly reported in individuals with anorexia nervosa and are thought to be related to altered gastric motility. Intestinal mucosa (i.e., the lining of the gastrointestinal tract) often becomes increasingly thin and smooth, caus-ing a decrease in the production of various digestive enzymes (e.g., lactase, sucrase, maltase, and aminopeptidase; Bo-Linn 1986; Carney and Andersen 1996). The result is a significant impairment of digestion and absorption of what little food is consumed, thereby further exacerbating the nutritionally deficient state. Mild to moderate lactose intolerance may develop because of the decrease in synthesis and activity of the enzyme lactase.

The compromised intestinal mucosa resulting from semistarvation may also increase the risk of stomach or peptic ulcers (Carney and Andersen 1996; De Caprio, Pasanisi, and Contaldo 2000). Certain habits common in those with anorexia nervosa—frequent or excessive gum chewing, coffee drinking, and sucking on hard candy—may contribute to increased acid production and heighten ulcer risk. The risk might be further exacerbated in athletes who also consume large amounts of anti-inflammatory medications. Finally, in cases of large and rapid weight loss, gallstones are a possibility (Carney and Andersen 1996).

Endocrine Abnormalities

Severe and/or chronic energy restriction has the potential to impair the function of a number of different endocrine glands, including the thyroid, adrenal, and pituitary glands. The overt effects of these glandular impair-ments are hormonal abnormalities, menstrual dysfunction in women, and testosterone suppression in men.

Hormonal Abnormalities

As previously mentioned, low levels of the active thyroid hormone, triiodo-thyronine (T3), are frequently seen in individuals who severely and/or chroni-cally restrict energy intake (Curran-Celentano et al. 1985; Gold et al. 1986). Overt symptoms of this low-T3 syndrome are similar to those associated with hypothyroidism and include fatigue, constipation, and cold intolerance.

Elevated plasma and cerebrospinal levels of cortisol are also common in individuals who severely and/or chronically restrict energy intake (Eichner 1992). Prolonged hypercortisolism can result in muscle wasting, decreased bone mineral density, and impaired immune function (McLean, Barr, and Prior 2001). In addition, since cortisol stimulates the secretion of stomach acid, chronically high levels of the hormone may increase the risk of stomach ulcers (Brook and Marshal 1996).

Menstrual Dysfunction

Menstrual dysfunction is a general term used to describe a variety of menstrual disorders, including luteal phase deficiency, anovulation, and exercise-associated amenorrhea (Otis 1992; Otis et al. 1997; see table 6.2). Luteal phase deficiency is characterized by a shortened luteal phase of the menstrual cycle (between ovulation and menstruation), which may be accompanied by a prolonged follicular phase (between menstruation and ovulation); thus, the total cycle length remains relatively unchanged, which makes detection very difficult (Otis 1992; Warren and Shanmugan 2000). Luteal phase deficiency was first reported in runners (Shangold et al. 1979) and swimmers (Bonen et al. 1981) who demonstrated normal total cycle lengths but who, upon biochemical evaluation, were later shown to suffer significant reductions in progesterone production and decreases in luteal phases length. More recent research has confirmed this initial observation, showing that women engaged in intense, prolonged training (e.g., training for a marathon) are at risk for developing luteal phase deficiency (Bruno et al. 1995; Otis 1992).

Anovulation, an absence of ovulation, is characterized by abnormal menstrual cycle lengths ranging from very short cycles (<21 days) to overly long cycles (35-150 days). A prolonged length of time between cycles (>35 days) is generally referred to as *oligomenorrhea* (Otis 1992). Like luteal phase deficiency, anovulation is characterized by reduced progesterone secretion. Unlike luteal phase deficiency, however, anovulation is more overtly obvious because of the abnormal total cycle length, although many athletes are either unaware of its significance or choose to ignore it.

Exercise-associated amenorrhea is the most widely studied and potentially dangerous form of menstrual dysfunction seen in female athletes (Otis 1992). Two forms of exercise-associated amenorrhea have been described in the literature: primary amenorrhea (the absence of menstrual periods by age 16) and secondary amenorrhea (the absence of three or more consecutive menstrual periods; Otis 1992). As a diagnostic criterion for anorexia nervosa, amenorrhea is a clinical feature of the severe and chronic energy restriction that is characteristic of the disorder (APA 1994). Research suggests that amenorrhea is also prevalent among female athletes (Arena et al. 1995). In fact, secondary amenorrhea may afflict as many as 66% of female athletes (depending on the sport studied and the criteria used to define amenorrhea; Eichner, 1992). A female athlete who chronically or severely restricts energy intake is thus at even greater risk for menstrual dysfunction (Dueck, Manore, and Matt 1996).

While the reason for the high prevalence of menstrual dysfunction among female athletes (particularly those with disordered eating) is not completely understood, there is a growing body of evidence suggesting that it may be the result of chronic energy drain, that is, low energy intake combined with high energy expenditure (Dueck, Manore, and Matt 1996; Loucks, Verdun, and Heath 1998; Williams et al. 1995). The cessation of menstrual function could thus be viewed as an energy-conserving strategy to protect more

Table 6.2   Menstrual Dysfunction Categories and Their Health Consequences

Menstrual dysfunction	Definition	Health consequences
Primary amenorrhea (delayed menarche)	Absence of menstruation by age 16 in girls with secondary sex characteristics.	• Increased risk of scoliosis • Failure to reach peak bone mass • Increased risk of premature osteoporosis
Secondary amenorrhea	Absence of three or more consecutive menstrual periods after menarche.	• Infertility problems • Decreased bone mineral density • Increased risk of musculoskeletal injuries (particularly stress fractures) • Increased risk of premature osteoporosis
Luteal phase deficiency	A shortened luteal phase, which may or may not be accompanied by a prolonged follicular phase. Progesterone production is significantly reduced, but total cycle length remains relatively unchanged.	• Possible precursor to secondary amenorrhea • Infertility problems • Decreased bone mineral density • Increased risk of musculoskeletal injuries (particularly stress fractures) • Increased risk of premature osteoporosis
Anovulation/ oligomenorrhea	The absence of ovulation combined with abnormal cycle lengths ranging from very short cycles (< 21 days) to overly long cycles (35-150 days). Prolonged cycle length is referred to as oligomenorrhea.	• May be a precursor to secondary amenorrhea • Infertility problems • Decreased bone mineral density • Increased risk of musculoskeletal injuries (particularly stress fractures) • Increased risk of premature osteoporosis

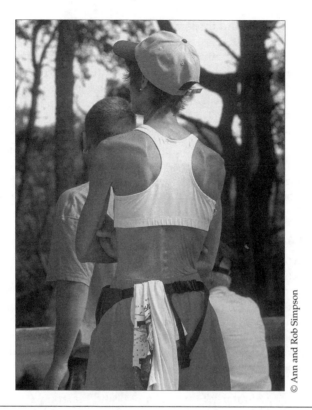

© Ann and Rob Simpson

Women engaged in prolonged, intense training are at risk of developing menstrual dysfunction, which can result in infertility, decreased immune function, lowered bone mass density, and a greater risk for premature osteoporosis.

important biological and reproductive processes. Indeed, a few studies show that energy deprivation can alter the hormonal profiles and subsequently the menstrual cycles of previously healthy women (Loucks, Verdun, and Heath 1998; Williams et al. 1995).

The extent of the menstrual dysfunction that occurs with energy restriction likely depends on at least three factors: (1) the degree of the energy restriction, (2) the body's level of energy reserves, and (3) the initial hormonal status before the energy restriction (Manore 1998). Thus, severe energy restriction is more likely to initiate menstrual dysfunction than mild energy restriction. Moreover, the combination of severe energy restriction and strenuous exercise undoubtedly has a larger negative impact on menstrual function than either energy restriction or exercise alone. This may be explained in part by the greater energy deficit and resulting weight loss that occurs when energy restriction is combined with high energy expenditure (Manore 1998). Similarly, menstrual dysfunction is more likely to occur in dieting athletes with low body weight or low body fat percentage (i.e., those with little weight or fat to lose) and those who have suffered some type of menstrual irregularity in the past.

Interestingly, female athletes who experience menstrual dysfunction, particularly amenorrhea, often demonstrate little concern for the disruption in their cycles; in fact, they often seem relieved by the "break." Similarly, some coaches simply dismiss menstrual dysfunction, believing it is simply a natural result of hard training. In fact, menstrual dysfunction is *not* a normal response to training; rather, it is a clear indication that health is being compromised. The health consequences of menstrual dysfunction are well documented and include infertility and other reproductive problems, decreased immune function, an increase in cardiovascular risk factors, and decreased bone mineral density and increased risk for premature osteoporosis (Constantini 1994).

Decreased Testosterone Levels

Depressed testosterone levels in male athletes may be the parallel of menstrual dysfunction in female athletes. That is, strenuous physical training combined with energy restriction may threaten men's reproductive function just as it does women's, resulting in a suppression of testicular function and thus temporary infertility. The limited available research seems to support this hypothesis. For example, Griffith et al. (1990) found that cyclists who abruptly increased their training load (i.e., by doubling their mileage) for a two-week period showed significant decreases in testosterone levels and sperm counts. They also reported feelings of fatigue, a decline in sex drive, and a reduction in sexual activity. Similarly, Strauss, Lanese, and Malarkey (1985) found low serum testosterone levels in male wrestlers who were actively cutting weight. Interestingly, testosterone levels in these wrestlers returned to normal during the off-season, when they regained the lost body weight.

As was the case with female athletes, the hormonal changes in male athletes who restrict energy intake are likely a function of the extent of the energy deficit incurred, the initial hormonal levels, and how far the athlete is below his normal body weight, although to date these hypotheses have not been tested.

Decreased Bone Mineral Density

Numerous studies have shown that females suffering from anorexia nervosa have reduced bone mineral density (BMD; Andersen, Woodward, and LaFrance 1995; Munoz and Argente 2002; Soyka et al. 1999; Ward, Brown, and Treasure 1997). If the reduction in BMD is more mild (i.e., between 1 and 2.5 standard deviations below the mean for age-matched individuals), it is referred to as osteopenia. More severe reductions in BMD (more than 2.5 standard deviations below the mean of age-matched individuals) are considered indicative of osteoporosis (Otis et al. 1997). The degree of BMD reduction seen with anorexia is generally considered to depend on three primary factors: (1) the degree of weight loss (particularly lean body mass),

(2) the length of time the disorder has persisted, and (3) the duration of amenorrhea (Castro et al. 2000; Schneider et al. 2002). Thus, the greater the weight loss (and loss of lean body mass) and the longer both anorexia and amenorrhea have persisted, the lower the BMD.

The persistent low body weight and abnormal hormonal profiles (i.e., depressed estrogen or androgen levels and elevated cortisol) character-istic of the athlete who severely or chronically restricts energy intake can together contribute to a reduction in BMD (osteopenia) that predisposes the athlete to musculoskeletal injuries (particular stress fractures) as well as premature osteoporosis (Constantini 1994; Drinkwater 1992; Myburgh et al. 1990; Otis et al. 1997). Indeed, research indicates that lumbar BMD can be reduced by as much as 20% in amenorrheic athletes compared with that in eumenorrheic athletes (Drinkwater et al. 1984, 1986; Marcus et al. 1985; Wolman et al. 1990). Moreover, the decrease in BMD may be partially irreversible despite resumption of normal menses, estrogen replacement, and/or calcium supplementation (Drinkwater et al. 1984, 1986; Drinkwater 1992). A series of landmark studies conducted in the mid-1980s by Barbara Drinkwater demonstrates the debilitating and last-ing effects of amenorrhea on bone health in female athletes (Drinkwater et al. 1984, 1986). In the first study the BMDs of 14 amenorrheic athletes were compared with those of 14 eumenorrheic athletes matched by age, height, weight, sport, and training regimen (Drinkwater et al. 1984). The amenorrheic athletes had significantly lower (approximately 14%) BMD at the lumbar vertebrae compared with the eumenorrheic athletes. For the second study, 16 of the original 28 athletes (9 amenorrheic and 7 eumen-orrheic) were followed for a total of three years, during which time 7 of the amenorrheic athletes regained menses (Drinkwater et al. 1986). The mean BMD for the two athletes who remained amenorrheic continued to decline (–3.4%), while the BMD for the eumenorrheic athletes remained relatively unchanged. The average BMD for the amenorrheic athletes who regained menses increased significantly (about 6%) during the first year; however, the increase slowed to only 3% the following year and then ceased altogether the year after that.

This study and others that have followed clearly show that the loss of BMD in athletes suffering from amenorrhea cannot be completely regained (Drinkwater 1992). This means that athletes with a history of amenorrhea will always have BMDs below (by as much as 20%) aged-matched, eumenorrheic controls and be at increased risk for musculoskeletal injuries (most notably stress fractures) and premature osteoporosis (Drinkwater, Bruemmer, and Chestnut 1990). Research has also shown that the osteopenia resulting from anorexia frequently persists even after recovery from the disease, despite restoration of body weight and normal menses (Munoz and Argente 2002; Ward, Brown, and Treasure 1997). Taken together, these findings indicate that the amenorrheic athlete who severely or chronically restricts energy intake is at a particularly high risk for osteopenia (and perhaps premature osteo-porosis) and all the musculoskeletal complications that accompany it.

No research to date has examined the effect of disordered eating on the BMD of male athletes. Nonetheless, limited research shows that male nonathletes suffering from anorexia nervosa experience decreases in BMD and are at increased risk for premature osteoporosis (Andersen, Gray, and Holman 1996; Andersen, Watson, and Schlechte 2000; Castro et al. 2002). For example, Castro et al. (2002) examined the BMDs of 20 male adolescents with anorexia nervosa and found that 35% ($n = 7$) had osteopenia and that duration of illness was significantly negatively correlated to BMD. Similarly, Andersen, Watson, and Schlechte (2000) analyzed the BMDs of 31 male patients at an eating disorders treatment center and found that 35% ($n = 11$) suffered from osteopenia. Moreover, in a number of cases the bone loss was significantly more severe than that seen in women with anorexia. Based on this data it would be safe to assume that the male athlete who severely and chronically restricts energy intake and maintains an abnormally low body weight is compromising his bone health as well.

Psychological Stress

In the classic study *The Biology of Human Starvation*, Ancil Keys and colleagues (1950) documented the deleterious effects of severe and chronic energy restriction combined with high levels of energy expenditure on the psyche of the starving individual. The experiment was designed to mimic the starvation seen in war-torn European countries after World War II. The results were intended to prepare aiding nations for the challenge of helping survivors and prisoners of war. For six months, 32 male volunteers consumed a protein- and energy-deficient diet (about 1,570 kcal/d, or half their habitual intake) and engaged in vigorous exercise combined with hard manual labor. As the energy-deprivation period progressed (and more and more weight was lost), the men grew increasingly weak, depressed, self-centered, and apathetic. They lost interest in almost everything—everything, that is, except food. When it came to food, their interest grew to the point of obsession. The men reported extreme food preoccupation; they would spend their days thinking about food and their nights dreaming about food. They also became extremely protective of their food and would hoard it at mealtimes; many reported secretly stowing away food for later consumption. As starvation ensued, the men also became increasingly socially isolated, withdrawing from individuals with whom they had previously shared friendships. Six of the men developed character neuroses, while two others developed mild psychoses (Keys et al. 1950).

If we relate these experiences to those of the athlete who severely or chronically restricts energy intake, we can begin to understand the psychological stress that he or she must endure. To be sure, the stress of continually denying hunger, obsessing about food, agonizing over body weight, and fearing weight gain must be mentally exhausting. With the mind so preoccupied with food, there is apt to be little time to think about anything else. Moreover, this preoccupation likely interferes with the athlete's performance of daily functions (e.g., handling interpersonal relationships, working, studying) as well as his or her training and competition.

Health Effects of Bingeing and Purging

Many of the health effects of bingeing and purging are similar to those of severe and/or chronic energy restriction, including endocrine abnormalities, decreased bone mineral density, and psychological stress. The gastrointestinal and cardiovascular complications resulting from bingeing and purging behaviors, however, are somewhat distinct from those associated with severe energy restriction. The unique effects of bingeing and purging on the health of the athlete are described in the following sections.

Gastrointestinal Disorders

Gastrointestinal disorders are common among individuals who regularly binge and purge. Bingeing generally results in gastric distention, the severity of which increases with an increase in the amount of food consumed during the binge. In rare cases, excessive bingeing can cause gastric necrosis and even rupture (Pomeroy and Mitchell 1992). Esophageal reflux is frequently experienced, particularly after late-night binges, as the contents of the engorged stomach create great intragastric pressure and allow the stomach contents to back up into the esophagus (Bo-Linn 1986; Carney and Andersen 1996). Individuals who use self-induced vomiting to purge also suffer frequent throat irritation and may be at increased risk of developing dental caries because of erosion of the tooth enamel (Carney and Andersen 1996).

Self-induced vomiting is the most widely used purging technique and can have profound consequences on the gastrointestinal tract. The frequency and severity of the vomiting, the composition of the gastric contents being regurgitated, and the age of the individual all play a role in the severity of the gastrointestinal complications (Carney and Andersen 1996). Recurrent vomiting of the acidic contents of the stomach can result in painful inflammation of the esophagus and esophageal ulcers (Bo-Linn 1986). Forceful vomiting can also cause tears (known as Mallory-Weis tears) and bleeding in the esophagus, and in extreme cases the esophagus can actually rupture (Pomeroy and Mitchell 1992).

A number of techniques are used to induce vomiting. An individual may use a finger or hand at the back of the throat to activate the gag reflex and induce vomiting. Some individuals who are unable or unwilling to induce vomiting manually take ipecac, an over-the-counter antidote for accidental poisoning. Frequent use of this product has been linked to severe and irreversible cardiac and skeletal muscle damage (Pomeroy and Mitchell 1992).

Laxative abuse is second only to self-induced vomiting as a purging technique, despite the fact that it is ineffective in ridding the body of consumed calories (associated with a binge) or inducing body fat loss (Carney and Andersen 1996). Gastrointestinal complications associated with laxative abuse include chronic diarrhea, severe abdominal cramping, irritation of the lining of the large intestine, and hemorrhoids (Bo-Linn 1986). Chronic use of laxatives can also disrupt the normal muscular action (i.e., peristalsis) of the large intestine, resulting in cathartic colon, a condition in which the colon becomes unable to function properly on its own (Pomeroy and Mitchell 1992). Thus, the individual grows increasingly dependent on laxatives to have a normal bowel movement. This is why breaking the laxative abuse cycle is often so difficult; cessation of use frequently leads to rebound constipation, gas, bloating, and severe abdominal cramping.

Electrolyte Imbalances

Electrolyte imbalances, particularly hypokalemia (i.e., low blood potassium levels), are common in individuals who engage in purging behaviors and can have debilitating effects on health. In fact, many of the deaths attributable to eating disorders are a direct result of electrolyte abnormalities (Bo-Linn 1986; Pomeroy and Mitchell 1992). While all the common purging methods (i.e., self-induced vomiting, laxatives, and diuretics) have the potential to induce electrolyte imbalances, the abuse of laxatives and

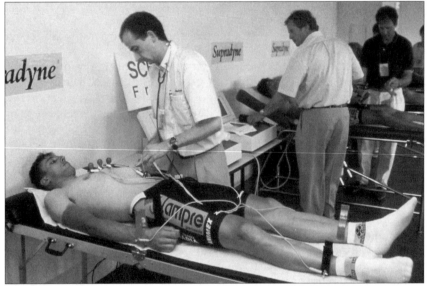

© Sport the Library

Complications of bingeing and purging that can be particularly detrimental to the athlete include electrolyte imbalances, cardiovascular complications, and disruptions of acid–base balance.

diuretics probably poses the greatest risk. Appetite suppressants and "fat burners" that contain caffeine, ephedrine, or other stimulants also act as mild diuretics and thus can promote electrolyte losses.

Hypokalemia causes disruptions in the heart's electrical impulses, which can lead to potentially fatal cardiac arrhythmia. Hypokalemia is particularly dangerous because it frequently occurs with few if any noticeable symptoms. While some individuals may experience heart palpitations, others are virtually asymptomatic, making it nearly impossible to predict when a life-threatening cardiac arrhythmia will occur (Carney and Andersen 1996; Pomeroy and Mitchell 1992). Diuretic abuse and/or self-induced vomiting leading to contraction alkalosis (abnormal elevations in the pH of the electrolyte mixture in extracellular fluid) can further complicate the problem by making the correction of potassium levels more difficult (Pomeroy and Mitchell 1992). Individuals with hypokalemia also tend to have underlying hypomagnesemia (low blood magnesium levels) and, less frequently, hyponatremia (low blood sodium levels; Carney and Andersen 1996).

Hyponatremia is also a potential complication of the purging behaviors and associated dehydration common in individuals with bulimia. It may be particularly problematic for the bulimic endurance athlete, as hyponatremia is most commonly seen during prolonged exercise events in which sweat losses and sodium losses are high (Noakes 2003). The calorie-conscious athlete may avoid food or sports drinks and consume nothing but water, resulting in a dilution of sodium in the plasma. Like hypokalemia, hyponatremia may be either symptomatic or asymptomatic. Symptoms, if they occur, include headache, nausea, vomiting, and epilepsy-like seizures (Noakes 2003).

Cardiovascular Changes

The cardiovascular complications associated with bingeing and purging are usually secondary to the electrolyte imbalances induced by purging. As described earlier, hypokalemia can result in potentially life-threatening cardiac arrhythmia. In addition, individuals who abuse ipecac may suffer myocarditis (inflammation of the middle layer of the heart muscle) and various cardiomyopathies (Carney and Andersen 1996).

Disruption of Acid–Base Balance

Alterations in electrolyte levels as a result of purging can lead to dangerous disruptions in the body's acid–base balance and life-threatening alterations in the body's pH. Self-induced vomiting typically results in an increase in serum bicarbonate levels and thus leads to metabolic alkalosis (increase in blood pH). On the other hand, individuals who abuse laxatives are most likely to develop metabolic acidosis (decrease in blood pH) secondary to loss of bicarbonate in the stool (Carney and Andersen 1996).

Summary

Many athletes believe that disordered eating practices are of little consequence to both their immediate and long-term health. On the contrary, severe and/or chronic energy restriction, bingeing, and purging can result in serious medical complications, including nutrient deficiencies; fluid and electrolyte imbalances; endocrine abnormalities; menstrual dysfunction; irreversible bone loss; and potentially fatal damage to the cardiovascular, metabolic, immune, and gastrointestinal systems. Athletes suffering from disordered eating must be made to understand and appreciate the dangers that their dieting practices can have on their health and performance.

The medical complications associated with disordered eating are likely to become increasingly severe the longer the disorder continues. Thus, it is imperative that coaches, athletic trainers, team physicians, and athletic support staff be able to recognize the signs and symptoms of disordered eating and have a plan of action for its medical management.

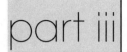

part iii

Managing Disordered Eating in Athletes

seven

Prevention of Disordered Eating in Athletes

CHAPTER OBJECTIVES

After reading this chapter, you will be able to

■ describe the importance of preventing disordered eating in athletes and

■ describe the components of educational programming for the prevention of disordered eating in athletes.

The previous two chapters clearly demonstrated that disordered eating behaviors can have severe and potentially long-lasting consequences on an athlete's health and performance. Furthermore, both scientific and anecdotal evidence suggest that treating eating disorders in athletes is a difficult, lengthy, and often ineffective process (see chapter 9 for more on treatment issues). It is for these reasons that *prevention* is considered the key to reducing disordered eating in athletes.

This chapter presents strategies for preventing disordered eating in athletes. Educational programs for athletes, coaches, and other athletic support staff are described. In addition, strategies are outlined for promoting healthful eating behaviors while at the same time moderating or even eliminating behaviors conducive to the development of disordered eating.

An Ounce of Prevention

According to Thompson and Sherman (1993), two well-known psychologists specializing in the treatment of eating disorders in athletes, the goal of eating disorder prevention is to inoculate athletes against the factors that predispose them to developing eating disorders. Such inoculation necessitates identifying the risk factors of disordered eating and then trying to eliminate or at least modify those risks. Unfortunately, as was shown in chapter 3, many of the factors that predispose an athlete to develop disordered eating (e.g., biological or psychological predisposition; dysfunctional family life; being female, Caucasian or of adolescent age) can be considered unalterable and as such are largely outside the control of coaches, athletic staff, or health professionals. Prevention efforts must therefore focus on those predisposing factors that can be controlled, that is, the sociocultural emphasis on thinness, unrealistic body weight ideals, and unhealthy eating and weight control practices that permeate the athletic environment.

Changing the way in which society as a whole views ideal of body weight and shape is a tall order and likely beyond the capabilities of athletic personnel or health professionals. Nonetheless, both athletic personnel and health professionals *can* help modify body weight or shape perceptions and expectations within the athletic environment and promote safe and sound nutritional practices. These goals are best accomplished by a combination of educational programs and preventive strategies.

Educational Programs

Educational programming for the prevention of disordered eating in athletes should target coaches, trainers, athletic support staff and administration, and the athletes themselves. The aim of educational efforts should be dispelling the myths and misconceptions surrounding nutrition, body weight and composition, weight loss, and the impact of these factors on athletic performance. Equally important is providing accurate and appropriate nutritional information and dietary guidelines to promote optimal health and athletic performance.

Nutrition and Athletic Performance

Research consistently shows that when it comes to nutrition, both athletes and athletic personnel (i.e., coaches, trainers, athletic administrators) lack sufficient knowledge. Moreover, much of the nutrition knowledge they do possess is derived from anecdotal reports and hearsay (i.e., advice from peers, dietary practices of successful athletes, and sports magazines; Chapman et al. 1997; Corley, Menarest-Litchford, and Bazzarre 1990; Jacobson, Sobonya, and Ransone 2001; Schmalz 1993; Smith-Rockwell, Nickols-Richardson, and Thye 2001). Lack of sound nutrition information combined with an abundance of misinformation may increase an athlete's risk for developing disordered eating behaviors. Some of the more common nutrition myths and misconceptions held by athletes suffering from disordered eating along with educational strategies to dispel them are described in the following paragraphs.

Athletes suffering from disordered eating frequently demonstrate a fear of not only body fat but also dietary fat. In fact, they often view the two as inseparable, harboring the belief that dietary fat will make them fat; thus, they maintain that fat must be eliminated from the diet (Beals and Manore 1998). In their misguided attempt to avoid dietary fat, some athletes rigidly swear off whole groups of foods, including meats and meat substitutes (e.g., peanut butter, beans, tofu), dairy products, and certain vegetables (e.g., olives, avocados, nuts). While eliminating these food groups will reduce dietary fat, it will also result in low intakes of protein, essential fatty acids, calcium, iron, and zinc, which can place athletes at risk for myriad health problems, not to mention impairing their performance (see chapters 5 and 6 for more on disordered eating, dieting, and athletic performance).

In addition to severely restricting dietary fat, an increasing number of athletes with disordered eating are restricting or eliminating carbohydrates from their diet (Beals and Manore 1998). Like the general dieting public, athletes seeking weight loss are being lured in by the low-carbohydrate diet programs' claims that carbohydrates not only promote weight gain but also inhibit weight loss and thus must be severely restricted or completely eliminated from the diet. Not surprisingly, these claims have not been supported by scientific research, nor have these diets been shown to be effective for long-term weight loss in clinical trials. Moreover, these diets can cause a variety of negative side effects (e.g., fatigue, glycogen depletion, hypoglycemia, dehydration, electrolyte imbalances), which may be little more than a nuisance for a sedentary dieter but can spell disaster for a competitive athlete. As described in chapter 5, carbohydrates are the primary fuel used by the body during exercise. Failure to provide the body with sufficient carbohydrate results in glycogen depletion and premature fatigue during exercise.

Finally, athletes with disordered eating often restrict fluid or voluntarily induce dehydration via the use of diuretics, saunas, and/or rubber suits to promote rapid weight loss. They are either unaware of or unconcerned by the fact that the weight loss is almost exclusively body water (not body fat) and that dehydration can have severe consequences on both health and athletic performance (see chapter 5 for more on dehydration and athletic performance). For these athletes, all that really matters is that the number on the scale has gone down.

Given the common myths and misconceptions described, nutrition education for the prevention of disordered eating in athletes should focus on the essential elements of a healthful diet, one that optimizes both training and competition. Because fat phobia seems to permeate the athletic arena, special attention should be given to the importance of consuming adequate amounts of dietary fat (at least 10% of energy intake) and the essential fatty acids. Nutrition education should highlight the different types of fats (i.e., saturated, monounsaturated, and polyunsaturated), their food sources, and their physiological and biochemical roles. Examples of lower-fat (and lower-saturated-fat) alternatives should be provided (e.g., low-fat dairy products, poultry, fish, and lean meats).

Nutrition education should also stress the importance of adequate dietary carbohydrate for optimal performance, dispel the low-carbohydrate diet myths, and provide suggestions for the selection, preparation, and timing (i.e., before, during, and after exercise) of carbohydrate-rich meals. Information regarding the different types of carbohydrates (simple vs. complex; refined vs. unrefined) and the roles that they play in the athlete's diet may also be useful. (See appendix D for low-fat, high-carbohydrate food selections.) Finally, the importance of proper hydration, the consequences of dehydration, and the specific guidelines for fluid replacement before, during, and after exercise should be discussed in detail. The American College of Sports Medicine (Convertino et al. 1996) has published a position statement outlining fluid replacement guidelines. In addition, the Gatorade Sports Science Institute maintains a comprehensive Web site full of scientific articles and informational handouts on fluid replacement (www.gssiweb.com) and have recently released a complete packet of educational materials (video, handouts, etc.), titled "Beat the Heat," for athletic personnel and health professionals.

Almost as important as what educational information is provided is who provides the information. It is very important that nutrition education be provided by a qualified nutrition professional, ideally a registered dietitian who specializes in the area of sport nutrition. A reasonable scenario would be for each athlete to receive two individual nutritional consultations with a registered dietitian, one at the beginning of the season to assess and address nutritional risks and one during the season to monitor nutritional progress. Individual consultations also provide an excellent opportunity to assess the athlete for risk factors, signs, and symptoms of disordered eating. Unfortunately, this kind of one-on-one nutritional consultation is not always readily available to athletes, in which case group or team consultations may be conducted. Team consultations should include a discussion of basic nutritional principles as well as the specific nutritional requirements of the sport being addressed. The effects of unhealthy dietary practices on health and performance should also be stressed.

Body Weight, Body Composition, and Athletic Performance

One of the most widely held misconceptions that continues to pervade the athletic environment (despite a lack of scientific evidence to support it), is that reducing body weight invariably leads to improved athletic performance. No one would dispute that an extreme or unhealthful excess of body weight (particularly if the excess weight is predominantly fat) can negatively impact athletic performance. But that does not necessarily mean that a lower body weight is always more advantageous (Wilmore 1992).

There are some sports in which excess body mass may actually enhance performance. For instance, physical activities that require the application of force, particularly against an external object (e.g., throwing, pushing, weightlifting), are positively related to absolute body weight and size (Houtkooper 2000). Thus, a defensive linebacker, powerlifter, or hammer thrower can actually benefit from greater body mass. On the other hand, there are some sports in which it would seem advantageous, at least from a strictly physiological standpoint, to maintain a lower body weight. These include sports that involve running (middle- and long-distance running, hockey, basketball), jumping (basketball, hurdling, volleyball, high jump, long jump, pole vault), or rotation of the body around an axis (gymnastics and diving; Houtkooper 2000; Williams 2001; Wilmore 1992). For these sports, extra weight is thought to be detrimental because it increases the mass or inertia of the athlete and, particularly in the case of excess fat, does not contribute directly to energy production. Thus, the extra weight theoretically reduces movement economy and increases energy demand, both of which will negatively impact performance (Williams 2001).

Despite the logic of this hypothesis, there is surprisingly little scientific evidence to support the notion that being thinner will always lead to improvements in the performance of sports involving running, jumping, and tumbling. For this reason, it should be stressed to athletes, coaches, and athletic staff that body weight is only one of many factors that affect physical performance and thus should not be overemphasized. Moreover, in some cases, weight loss or the maintenance of an extremely low body weight may create more problems for the athlete than being a few pounds overweight. For example, an already lean athlete is not likely to derive any additional benefits from weight loss. On the contrary, weight loss for this athlete will probably lead to both performance and health decrements, particularly if the weight loss is too rapid or consists of a significant amount of lean body mass. Similarly, weight loss is unlikely to improve the performance of anaerobic

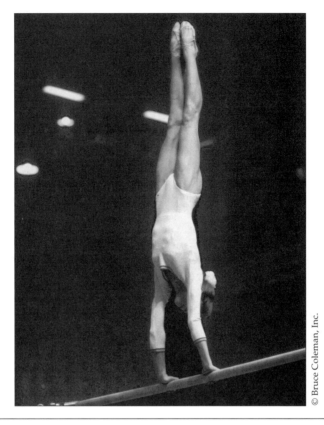

© Bruce Coleman, Inc.

Eating disorder prevention efforts must focus on the predisposing factors that can be controlled, including unrealistic body weight ideals as well as unhealthy eating and weight control practices that permeate the athletic environment.

or strength athletes (e.g., football players, gymnasts, and divers) or those in sports that do not require the body to move against gravity (e.g., cyclists and swimmers). Finally, any reduction in weight that is accomplished by severe energy restriction or pathogenic weight control techniques is likely to lead to decrements, not improvements, in athletic performance as well as increases in illnesses and injuries (Houtkooper 2000). (See chapters 5 and 6 for effects of disordered eating on athletic performance and health.)

Realizing the inaccuracies and potential dangers associated with body weight assessment, many coaches and trainers are replacing the measurement of body weight with that of body composition or body fat percentage (Skinner and Grooms 2002; Williams 2001). This, however, may be akin to "coming out of the frying pan and into the fire." That is, while various researchers have reported body fat percentages of successful athletes in specific sports, there is currently no data to indicate that body composition by itself predicts athletic performance (Houtkooper 2000). Moreover, as with any indirect anthropometric measurement, a margin of error is involved. For most body composition measurements, the error rate can range from 3% to 6%. Thus, an athlete who actually has 15% body fat could have a predicted value as high as 21% or as low as 9%. Finally, for some athletes the assessment of body composition can be equally if not more traumatic as the measurement of body weight and, thus, has the potential to cause body image disturbances and disordered eating behaviors in vulnerable athletes.

Because the psychological and physiological costs of body weight or composition measurements can outweigh any potential benefits, some athletic organizations are calling for the elimination of these and other anthropometric measurements. For example, the Canadian Academy of Sport Medicine has recently issued a position statement calling for the abandonment of routine body composition assessment in female athletes (Carson and Bridges 2001). Several other national sports and medical organizations have suggested that both weigh-ins and body composition assessments be eliminated or at the very least be used with extreme caution (Otis et al. 1997).

Unfortunately, in many sport settings, eliminating anthropometric assessments may not be a viable or even the most appropriate solution. There are instances when anthropometric measurements may be valuable. For example, body composition measurements taken at regular intervals throughout an athlete's season can help in evaluating the efficacy of a given training program, monitoring the effects of dietary changes, and identifying any unusual or unhealthy weight fluctuations. In the case of an athlete with a known eating disorder, monitoring body weight or composition is essential to ensure that the athlete is following the treatment plan and adhering to his or her guidelines. Finally, for young athletes, anthropometric measurements are important for evaluating appropriate growth and maturation (Skinner and Grooms 2002). If anthropometric assessments are utilized, however, they should be conducted by a qualified health professional (preferably not the coach) who can thoughtfully and objectively interpret and communicate the results to the athlete.

Athletes need to fully understand why the measurements are being taken and what the results mean in terms of health and performance (Ryan 1992a). In addition, athletes should be informed of the potential sources of error in the measurement used and the limitations of body composition assessment in general. When evaluating body composition, an athlete's measurements should not be compared with standardized norms nor with those of other athletes. Rather, body composition assessment should be used only to monitor an athlete's own changes over the season, to chart an individual athlete's training progress, or to evaluate the effectiveness of a dietary regimen or training program. The athlete and the health professional should work together to formulate a body composition goal, keeping in mind the athlete's body size, shape, and structure as well as his or her weight and body composition history (see the sidebar; Skinner and Grooms 2002).

How Should Ideal Body Weight Be Defined?

Ideal body weight has been defined in numerous ways by a variety of researchers and practitioners. Generally, it is defined as a given weight for height or, more recently, as a body fat percentage that is associated with minimal disease risk (or in the case of athletes, a body fat percentage typical for a given sport). Yet the normative values that are frequently used for body weight and body composition do not take into account individual differences in body size, structure, and shape. There is no chart or table that can accurately determine each individual athlete's ideal body weight or body composition. Thus, some alternative definitions of ideal body weight or composition have been suggested (Manore and Thompson 2000):

- A body weight or composition that is relatively easily maintained. The achievement and maintenance of an ideal body weight or composition should not have to rely on stringent dieting and excessive exercise. Rather, it should be one that the athlete can achieve and maintain while consuming a healthful diet and engaging in adequate amounts of physical activity.

- A body weight or composition that allows adequate nutrition. It should allow the consumption of an adequate number of calories and the intake of all essential vitamins and minerals. If energy intake has to be limited to under 1,000 kcal/d to achieve the body weight, then it is *not* the ideal weight.

- A body weight or composition that is associated with optimal health (or minimal risk of disease). Excess body weight or body fat can increase the risk for disease, but so can a body weight or percentage of body fat that is too low. The ideal body weight or composition affords the athlete optimal health and well-being.

- A body weight or composition that allows optimal performance in the chosen sport. The ideal body weight or composition for an athlete in a given sport is very difficult to determine. In general, a higher ratio of lean body mass to fat mass is associated with better performance in most sports; however, too little body fat results in deterioration of health and performance.

- A body weight or composition that is individualized. It should take into consideration the athlete's genetic makeup, family history of body weight and body shape, and the athlete's body size and structure.

Ideally, neither the coach nor other athletic support staff should have any direct involvement in body weight or composition assessment of the athlete. Nonetheless, even if they are not directly involved, all athletic personnel should receive appropriate education in the area of anthropometric assessment. This includes information on the limitations and sources of error inherent in anthropometric measurements and the physiological consequences of a body weight or body fat percentage that is either too low or too high. In addition, all athletic personnel should be made aware of the psychological impact that anthropometric assessments can have on the athlete (e.g., the potential stress such measurements can cause the athlete and the potential for initiating or exacerbating disordered eating behaviors). Last but not least, coaches, trainers, and other athletic staff must remember to keep body composition measurements in perspective, understanding that body composition is not a primary determinant of athletic success (Williams 2001).

Dieting, Weight Loss, and Athletic Performance

The myths and misinformation surrounding dieting, weight loss, and athletic performance likely rival those regarding body weight, body composition, and nutrition. As mentioned previously, many coaches and athletes believe that weight loss, *by any means,* will invariably lead to improvement in performance. Again, the evidence (discussed in chapter 5), both scientific and anecdotal, does not support this notion.

This is not to say, however, that weight loss is *never* appropriate for an athlete. There are certain circumstances when weight loss or, more specifically, fat loss may be warranted (e.g., when a significant decrement in performance accompanies a significant increase in body weight or body fat). When there is sufficient evidence that weight or fat loss could prove beneficial to athletic performance, the athlete should be referred to a health or nutrition professional (preferably the team physician or sport dietitian), who can provide the appropriate dietary strategies for achieving safe and permanent weight loss.

Unfortunately, athletes do not always have access to a health professional who is sufficiently trained in weight management. In fact, more often than not, it is the coach or athletic trainer to whom the athlete turns for weight control advice. Thus, coaches, trainers, and the athletes themselves can benefit from education regarding proper methods of weight control. The educational program should emphasize the dangers associated with severe energy restriction and pathogenic weight loss methods while providing the basic guidelines for safe and effective weight or fat loss (Otis et al. 1997). (For advice on safe weight loss, go to www.eatright.org or www.gssiweb.com.)

Menstrual Dysfunction and Athletic Performance

It is both surprising and disconcerting how little female athletes seem to know about the menstrual cycle. Many do not realize the importance of their monthly cycle to overall health and athletic performance (Otis and Goldingay 2000). As mentioned in chapter 6, many female athletes view disruptions or even complete cessation of their cycles as a welcomed break (Otis and Goldingay 2000). Similarly, many coaches are unaware of the dangers that menstrual dysfunction can pose to the athlete's health and performance. Indeed, some coaches believe that menstrual dysfunction is a normal adaptation to training, and a few even continue to view it as a sign of peak condition (Otis and Goldingay 2000). Still others maintain a "don't ask, don't tell" policy regarding their athletes' menstrual function. They may feel uncomfortable discussing the issue with their athletes, or they may simply not view it as a significant aspect of health or performance.

As described in chapter 6, menstrual dysfunction can contribute to myriad health problems for the athlete, including infertility, decreased immune function, reduced bone mineral density, increased risk for musculoskeletal injuries, and premature osteoporosis. Moreover, because menstrual dysfunction is often a result of energy imbalance, it could very well be a sign of disordered eating. Thus, at the very least, coaches and trainers need to know if an athlete is experiencing menstrual dysfunction and ideally be privy to the type of menstrual dysfunction the athlete is experiencing (e.g., amenorrhea, oligomenorrhea). If a coach or trainer is uncomfortable discussing menstrual dysfunction with his or her athletes, female athletes should be referred to an appropriate health professional, such as a team physician, nurse practitioner, or a registered dietitian who specializes in female athletes, who can evaluate the athlete's menstrual function and provide recommendations for treatment of any dysfunction or irregularities.

Prevention Strategies

Any behaviorist would likely attest to the fact that increasing knowledge alone is not likely to change behavior. Thus, while education is certainly an important part of any eating disorder prevention program, it is unlikely to be effective unless it is accompanied by preventive efforts designed to change the beliefs and behaviors of athletes and athletic staff. The prevention strategies employed should build on the educational information supplied and thus should focus on de-emphasizing body weight and body composition, promoting healthful eating behaviors, destigmatizing disordered eating, and recognizing and encouraging the athlete's individuality while also fostering a team environment.

De-emphasize Weight and Body Composition

Emphasizing weight or body fat can cause the athlete to develop body dissatisfaction, which may in turn lead to disordered eating behaviors or the use of pathogenic weight control methods (Skinner and Grooms 2002). Thus, taking the emphasis off body weight and composition seems to be a logical first step toward preventing disordered eating behaviors in athletes. There are a number of ways that coaches, trainers, and athletic staff can help to de-emphasize body weight and composition among their athletes. As mentioned in the previous section, simply educating the athletes and athletic staff about the limitations of anthropometric measurements can help to reduce the emphasis placed on body weight and composition (or at least put it into proper perspective). Of course, the most obvious way to de-emphasize body weight or composition is to eliminate anthropometric assessments.

Routine weigh-ins, whether in a group setting or individually, do little more than create unneeded stress for the athlete and strain between the athlete and coach. Similarly, body composition assessment, although frequently viewed by health professionals and athletic personnel as a more accurate measure, is often viewed by athletes, particularly those suffering from disordered eating, as just another unattainable standard that can deliver quite a blow to their body image and self-esteem.

For these reasons, then, both body weight and body composition measurements should be eliminated from the athletic setting unless a health professional can provide sufficient rationale for their necessity. If there truly is a valid reason why body weight or body composition should be measured, then the measurement should be done in a private setting by someone other than the coach, such as the team physician, athletic trainer, registered dietitian, nurse, exercise physiologist, or other qualified health professional. In some cases it may be appropriate to withhold the results of the body weight or composition assessment from the athlete (e.g., if he or she is suffering from disordered eating and is anxious about weight gain or obsessive about weight loss). If the athletic staff does not make weight an issue, chances are the athletes won't either.

Promote Healthful Eating Behaviors

To successfully promote healthful eating behaviors among athletes, nutrition education and information must be reinforced by practice. All those involved in the management of athletes must then practice what they preach. Coaches are probably in the best position to reinforce nutrition education messages. (Unfortunately, they can also easily undermine them!)

For example, if athletes are taught about healthful eating and provided information on food choices to optimize performance but the coach does not make healthful snacks available during workouts or takes the athletes to fast-food restaurants for pre- or postgame meals, this undermines the effectiveness of nutrition education. On the other hand, if the coach provides healthful snacks during workouts and seeks restaurants with healthful choices for team meals, this helps reinforce the nutrition education and encourages the adoption of healthful eating behaviors. The coach can also help reinforce nutrition education by modeling healthful eating habits him- or herself. Coaches should make special efforts to follow the nutritional guidelines presented during nutrition education sessions. Leading by example is a well-recognized method of eliciting desired behavior changes.

Destigmatize Disordered Eating

The educational campaigns and media attention given to disordered eating have certainly increased awareness. However, it has done little to lessen the associated stigma. Athletes suffering from disordered eating often feel ashamed of their disorder; they typically feel that they are weak and have somehow failed themselves and those close to them. Moreover, they frequently live in fear of discovery and of being ostracized by teammates, peers, and society in general. For these reasons, athletes with disordered eating are understandably reluctant to come forward and admit to their disorder. Thus, if we are to hope that athletes with disordered eating accept help willingly or seek treatment of their own accord, we must destigmatize disordered eating within the athletic environment.

Coaches, trainers, and other athletic personnel can help to reduce the stigma of disordered eating by creating an atmosphere in which athletes feel comfortable discussing their concerns regarding body image, eating, and weight control. Athletic personnel should strive to promote understanding and foster trust between themselves and their athletes. The goal is to create an atmosphere in which athletes feel comfortable confiding an eating problem. In short, coaches, trainers, and athletic administrators must make it clear that they place the athletes' health and well-being ahead of athletic performance.

Recognize and Encourage the Athlete's Individuality

Many athletes try to emulate the eating and dieting habits of athletes that they admire in the hopes of achieving a similar physique, competitive status, and degree of athletic success (i.e., they want to "be like Mike"). Similarly, coaches frequently ascribe to their athletes the dietary regimens and body weight standards of other successful athletes whom they have trained or heard about.

Most coaches and athletes have come to realize the importance of individualizing physical training regimens. They accept that each athlete has a unique set of needs when it comes to the type, intensity, and duration of training necessary for optimal performance. Thus, it is surprising that they find it difficult to accept that each athlete has a unique body size, shape, and composition with distinct nutritional requirements. When it comes to an athlete's body weight or composition and his or her nutritional needs, there is no "one size fits all." Every athlete is physiologically unique, and thus body weight or composition goals and dietary practices should be developed specifically for each athlete, taking into account his or her weight and nutritional history, current training and dietary practices, and weight, diet, and performance goals.

Just as important as acknowledging individual physiological and nutritional differences is respecting athletes' psychological and emotional differences (Thompson and Sherman 1993). Some athletes are likely to be more sensitive to comments or criticism regarding body weight or composition than others. A casual comment about excess body weight may be readily disregarded by some athletes, while for others it may be enough to induce disordered eating behaviors. Because it may be difficult to identify which athletes are vulnerable, all athletes should be treated with care when it comes to body weight, shape, and composition. Better yet, those who manage athletes should avoid discussing body weight or composition with the athlete altogether. Instead, the focus should be on healthful eating behaviors and dietary practices for optimal performance.

Foster a Team Environment

While it is important to recognize and respect the athlete's individuality, it is also important to foster a team environment, one in which all athletes work together toward the common goal of optimal health and performance. Unfortunately, this may not be as easy as it sounds, particularly when it comes to the issues of eating and body weight or composition. Athletes by their very nature are competitive, and this competitive drive sometimes goes beyond the playing field affecting other aspects of the athlete's existence, such as eating behaviors, body weight, or body composition. Comparing oneself physically to another individual is certainly not a practice confined to athletes. However, it may be more prevalent in the athletic setting simply because athletes have more opportunities for comparison (e.g., athletes frequently change clothes and shower in the same locker room, athletic apparel or uniforms are becoming increasingly revealing, group weigh-ins and body composition assessments remain prevalent in many sports).

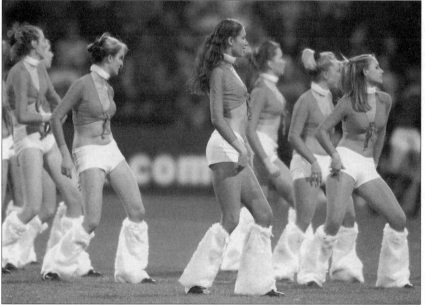

© Empics

Disordered eating may be fostered indirectly by the team environment, in which teammates sometimes observe and mimic disordered eating behaviors. This "contagion effect" may also explain the disparity in prevalence rates within different sports (e.g., thin-build sports such as dancing).

While it is probably not realistic to think that comparisons of body weight and composition between athletes can be eliminated, they certainly can and should be reduced. Coaches, trainers, and athletic administrators can help reduce "competitive thinness" by not comparing athletes' body weights or body compositions and by not using certain athletes on the team as the gold standard by which all others are measured. Instead, coaches and trainers should try to downplay body weight and encourage healthful eating behaviors among their athletes. The goal is to foster a team environment in which everyone works together toward a common goal of meeting energy and nutrient requirements.

A concern that has occasionally been expressed by athletic personnel and health care professionals is that the team environment might actually foster the development of disordered eating (Garner and Rosen 1991). It has been hypothesized that athletes might actually learn pathogenic weight control behaviors from teammates either directly by trading weight loss secrets or indirectly by observing and mimicking the behaviors of teammates with disordered eating. This "contagion effect" has been used to explain incidents of communal purging (e.g., wrestlers who dehydrate together, gymnasts who vomit together; Thompson and Sherman 1993) as well as the high prevalence rates of disordered eating in certain sports.

While it is true that athletes frequently turn to their teammates for training, eating, and even dieting advice, it does not necessarily follow that an athlete will "catch" an eating disorder from a teammate. As previously described, there are many factors that predispose an athlete to developing an eating disorder, few of which are exclusively impacted by the athletic environment. Thus, it is highly unlikely that disordered eating is simply a result of modeling behaviors. On the contrary, learning by example could actually prove beneficial in preventing disordered eating, so long as the behavior being modeled is one of healthful eating and safe weight control. Coaches, trainers, and other athletic personnel can help foster a suitable learning environment by making sure that their athletes receive appropriate and accurate nutrition education and by being very clear and direct about the acceptability of eating behaviors and weight loss practices.

A Final Word About Prevention

A number of studies have examined the efficacy of eating disorder prevention programs in the general population, and the results have been uniformly disappointing (Carter, Stewart, and Fairburn 1998; Killen et al. 1993; Mann et al. 1997; Paxton 1993). Specifically, the studies have demonstrated that, although program participants' knowledge increases, disordered eating *behaviors* are not reduced (and in some cases even increase). It should be emphasized that these studies were conducted largely on young, nonathletic women. To date, there has been no research examining the efficacy of eating disorder prevention programs in an athletic setting.

Until research suggests otherwise, eating disorder prevention should still be considered a priority in the athletic setting. Moreover, coaches, trainers, and athletic administrators must take an active role in the development and implementation of education and prevention programs for disordered eating (see the sidebar). In addition, whenever feasible, athletes should be consulted, if not directly involved, in the development and implementation of preventive programming (see chapter 11 for further discussion). The goal is to create feelings of ownership and confidence in prevention programs for disordered eating. If athletic personnel do not endorse education and prevention programs and if athletes cannot buy into the programs, they are unlikely to be successful.

Steps for Developing a Prevention Program

Dr. Randa Ryan, who developed and implemented one of the first and best-known eating disorder identification and prevention programs for female athletes, proposed a series of steps for developing intervention programs (Ryan 1992a). These same steps can be readily adapted to developing prevention strategies.

- Identify and isolate the predisposing factors within the specific athletic setting that can be altered (i.e., those factors thought to place the athlete at risk for developing disordered eating, such as unrealistic body weight ideals and unhealthful eating and weight control practices that often permeate the athletic environment).

- Develop educational materials and programs to address these predisposing factors.

- Create goals and develop a plan of action (i.e., preventive strategies) to combat these predisposing factors.

Summary

The key to reducing the incidence of disordered eating among athletes is to prevent disordered eating from developing in the first place. A two-pronged approach involving education and preventive efforts should be used. Education should focus on dispelling the myths and misconceptions surrounding nutrition, body weight or composition, weight loss, and their impact on performance while stressing the role of sound nutrition in promoting health and optimal performance. Preventive strategies in the athletic environment should be aimed at changing the prevailing misinformation, attitudes, and practices regarding nutrition, dieting, body weight or composition, and athletic performance that are too often an accepted part of sports.

eight

Identification of Disordered Eating in Athletes

CHAPTER OBJECTIVES

After reading this chapter, you will be able to

- describe the various techniques typically used to identify disordered eating in athletes,

- describe the eating disorder screening questionnaires currently available and identify their strengths and limitations,

- describe the structured interviews currently available for identifying disordered eating in athletes and identify their strengths and limitations, and

- list the warning signs and symptoms of disordered eating.

It was concluded in the previous chapter that the most effective way to reduce the incidence of eating disorders among athletes is to prevent them from occurring in the first place. While this may sound simple and straightforward on the surface, the previous chapter demonstrated that preventing the development of disordered eating among athletes is a complex and somewhat challenging task. Moreover, even the most comprehensive prevention program is not likely to be effective 100% of the time; thus, there will always be those athletes with disordered eating who slip through the cracks.

Throughout this book, it has been emphasized that the complications to health and performance associated with disordered eating and the treatment outcomes are related to the chronicity of the disorder. In other words, the longer the eating disorder is allowed to persist and progress without treatment, the greater the health and performance decrements and the more difficult it is to treat the disorder successfully. For these reasons, early identification is critical.

This chapter presents a description and evaluation of the currently available methods and instruments for identifying disordered eating among athletes. Because the most common methods of identification involve the use of questionnaires, a major focus of the chapter is describing these screening tools and evaluating their efficacy (or lack thereof).

Difficulty of Identification

Athletes suffering from disordered eating generally either deny that the problem exists or do not even realize that they have a problem. In either case they are unlikely to come forward and admit to disordered eating of their own accord. Thus, it is up to those who are close to the athlete (e.g., coaches, athletic trainers, peers, counselors, and parents) to recognize the signs and symptoms of disordered eating and initiate intervention. Unfortunately, too often the very individuals who are in the best position to identify athletes with disordered eating may unwittingly create barriers to that identification (Ryan 1992a). For example, coaches may choose to ignore or even dismiss the signs of disordered eating in their athletes because

- they may feel that they lack the knowledge, experience, or resources necessary to deal with the problem;
- they may not want to interfere with the success of an athlete who is training and performing well; or
- they may fear that they will be blamed for creating or contributing to the disordered eating behaviors.

Similarly, parents may inadvertently create barriers to identification out of a desire to see their child succeed (regardless of the consequences) or because they feel ill-equipped to deal with the disordered eating behaviors (Ryan 1992a). Teammates may be reluctant to identify a peer with disordered eating for fear of being labeled a "tattle-tale" or breaking the trust of a member of the team. They may also recognize that they too are suffering from disordered eating and fear that identifying a teammate will also implicate them (Ryan 1992a).

Of course, the athletes themselves, by virtue of their steadfast denial or lack of awareness of the problem, pose the greatest barrier (Ryan 1992a). Even those who have acknowledged their disordered eating are likely so besieged with guilt and shame that they will go to great lengths to conceal their problem. This makes identifying those with disordered eating difficult at best.

Unfortunately, there is currently no single fail-safe method or tool for identifying disordered eating in athletes. Instead, a combination of screening methods to identify disordered eating in athletes is considered the most successful approach. The most appropriate combination of screening methods depends on both the nature and dynamics of the athletic environment, the athletic staff, and the athletes themselves.

Screening

Screening for disordered eating in athletes is most often accomplished by using self-report questionnaires, personal interviews, or both. Unfortunately, most of the screening instruments available rely on athletes to self-report their disordered eating behaviors; thus, they are subject to response bias and distortion. Personal interviews probably provide a more accurate assessment of disordered eating in athletes; however, they must be both conducted and interpreted by a qualified professional. Moreover, the validity of personal interviews still depends on the athlete's answering the questions honestly and accurately. Some of the more common eating disorder screening questionnaires and interview instruments, as well as a newly developed instrument that shows great promise, are described in the following sections.

Self-Report Questionnaires

A number of surveys and questionnaires are available for screening athletes for disordered eating. Table 8.1 describes some of the most widely used instruments along with their strengths and limitations. Unfortunately, most of the instruments that have consistently been shown to be valid and reliable in the literature—such as the Eating Attitudes Test (EAT; Garner and Garfinkel 1979; Garner et al. 1982), Eating Disorder Inventory (EDI; Garner 1991; Garner, Olmstead, and Polivy 1983), and Bulimia Test Revised (BULIT-R; Thelen et al. 1991)—have not been validated in athletes and thus may not be appropriate for use in an athletic population. Conversely, those questionnaires that have been developed specifically for athletes—such as the Female Athlete Screening Tool (FAST; McNulty et al. 2001) and Athletic Milieu Direct Questionnaire (AMDQ; Nagel et al. 2000)—have not been sufficiently tested or validated in this population. In addition, administration and interpretation of many of the instruments necessitate a high degree of expertise or experience and may require interpretation by a qualified professional. For example, the Eating Disorder Inventory-2 can be purchased and

Table 8.1 Self-Report Surveys and Questionnaires for Identifying Disordered Eating in Athletes

Instrument	Description	Strengths	Limitations
Athletic Milieu Direct Questionnaire (AMDQ; Nagel et al. 2000)	A 19-item questionnaire designed to assess the clinical eating disorders (i.e., anorexia nervosa, bulimia nervosa, and eating disorders not otherwise specified) as well as disordered eating. The questionnaire assesses body image, dieting practices, and body weight changes as they relate to eating disorders and disordered eating. A variety of response categories are used, including a 4- to 6-point Likert scale, dichotomous response (yes or no), and multiple response.	• First instrument to operationalize the construct of disordered eating • Developed specifically to measure eating disorders and disordered eating in female athletes • Greater accuracy in identifying female athletes with eating disorders and disordered eating than either the EDI-2 or the BULIT-R	• May not be appropriate for male athletes • Has not been validated in a clinical population
Bulimia Test-Revised (BULIT-R; Thelen et al. 1991)	A 28-item multiple-choice questionnaire designed to assess the severity of symptoms and behaviors associated with bulimia nervosa (e.g., weight preoccupation and bingeing and purging frequency). Respondents rate each item on a 5-point Likert scale in which higher scores are more indicative of bulimia nervosa.	• Demonstrated validity (content, construct, and criterion) and reliability in both clinically identified bulimic patients and nonclinical college female populations	• Not specific to athletes • Not validated in an athletic population
Eating Attitudes Test, 40 items (EAT-40; Garner and Garfinkel 1979)	A 40-item inventory designed to assess thoughts, feelings, and behaviors associated with anorexia nervosa. Items are scored on a 6-point Likert scale ranging from *never* to *always*. A score of ≥30 indicates risk of anorexia nervosa.	• Valid in both clinical and nonclinical samples • Internal consistency reported to be high • Good test–retest reliability	• Not specific to athletes • Not validated in an athletic population

Eating Attitudes Test, 26 items (EAT-26; Garner et al. 1982)	A shortened (26-item) version of the EAT-40 that also identifies thoughts, feelings, and behaviors associated with anorexia nervosa. Uses a 6-point Likert scale ranging from *rarely* to *always*. A score of ≥20 indicates risk of anorexia nervosa.	• Valid and reliable in both clinical and nonclinical samples	• Not specific to athletes • Not validated in an athletic population
Eating Disorder Inventory (EDI; Garner, Olmstead, and Polivy 1983)	A 64-item questionnaire with 8 subscales. The first 3 subscales (Drive for Thinness, Bulimia, and Body Dissatisfaction) assess behaviors regarding body image, eating, and weight control practices. The remaining 5 subscales (Interpersonal Distrust, Perfectionism, Interoceptive Awareness, Maturity Fears, and Ineffectiveness) assess the various psychological disturbances characteristic of those with clinical eating disorders. Items are answered using a 6-point Likert scale ranging from *always* to *never*.	• Valid and reliable in both clinical and nonclinical samples	• Not specific to athletes • Not validated in an athletic population
Eating Disorder Inventory-2 (EDI-2; Garner 1991)	A 91-item multidimensional inventory designed to assess the symptoms of anorexia nervosa and bulimia nervosa. The EDI-2 contains the same 8 subscales as the EDI and adds 3 additional subscales (27 more items), including Asceticism, Impulse Regulation, and Social Insecurity. Items are answered using a 6-point Likert scale ranging from *always* to *never*.	• Test–retest reliability is good for short durations (<1 yr) • Shown to be valid in clinical samples	• Lower validity and reliability than the original EDI • Not specific to athletes • Not validated in an athletic population

(continued)

121

Table 8.1 *(continued)*

Instrument	Description	Strengths	Limitations
Female Athlete Screening Tool (FAST; McNulty et al. 2001)	A 33-item multiple-choice questionnaire specifically designed to identify disordered eating (e.g., "I think that being thin is associated with winning") and excessive exercise or exercise dependence (e.g., "If I cannot exercise, I find myself worrying that I will gain weight") in female athletes.	• Specific to female athletes and the athletic environment • Assesses excessive exercise, exercise dependence, and disordered eating	• May not be appropriate for male athletes • Not sufficiently validated in an athletic population
Survey of Eating Disorders Among Athletes (SEDA; Guthrie 1991)	A 33-item questionnaire that identifies self-reported eating pathology as well as factors specific to the athletic environment that may contribute to eating disorders.	• Developed and revised by professionals who work with athletes, students, and those with eating disorders	• Not sufficiently validated in an athletic population
Three-Factor Eating Questionnaire (TFEQ; Stunkard 1981)	A 58-item true/false and multiple-choice questionnaire that measures the tendency toward voluntary and excessive restriction of food intake as a means of controlling body weight. The questionnaire contains 3 subscales: Restrained Eating (e.g., "I often stop eating when I am not full as a conscious means of controlling my weight"), Tendency Toward Disinhibition (e.g., "When I feel lonely, I console myself by eating"), and Perceived Hunger (e.g., "I am always hungry enough to eat at any time").	• Good internal consistency and test–retest reliability • Adequate content and construct validity	• May not be appropriate for assessing disordered eating • Not specific to athletes • Not validated in an athletic population

used only by a licensed psychologist, psychiatrist, or equally qualified health professional. Thus, many of the currently available screening instruments may not be appropriate or even available to athletic personnel.

Finally, and perhaps most importantly, is the issue of *accuracy*. A questionnaire can function as an effective screening tool only if it provides an accurate assessment of the athlete's eating behaviors. This requires that the athlete not only interpret the questions correctly but also answer them truthfully. As the following studies demonstrate, these key requirements are probably not met as frequently as health professionals might think; thus, the validity and usefulness of most self-report questionnaires is highly questionable (O'Connor, Lewis, and Kirchner 1995; Sundgot-Borgen 1993b; Wilmore 1991).

A series of studies reported by Dr. Jack H. Wilmore (1991) clearly demonstrates the propensity for self-report questionnaires to miss substantial numbers of disordered eating cases. In the first study the EDI was used to assess eating disorders in a sample of 14 female distance runners. Only 3 of the 14 athletes were identified by the questionnaire as being at risk for disordered eating by the EDI. However, about one year later, 7 runners were diagnosed with and treated for an eating disorder (Wilmore 1991). In a second and somewhat similar study, the EAT was administered to 110 elite female athletes. Not a single athlete scored in the disordered eating range on the EAT, yet 18 were later diagnosed and treated for either anorexia or bulimia nervosa (Wilmore 1991).

In a more recent series of studies, O'Connor, Lewis, and Kirchner (1995) demonstrated how easy it is for athletes to answer incorrectly or deliberately falsify responses to eating disorder self-report questionnaires (such as the EDI) and how susceptible these instruments are to response distortion. In the first study, 21 college women completed the EDI-2 twice. The first time, the subjects were instructed to answer honestly, and the second time, they were told to answer dishonestly or fake their responses in a desirable fashion (i.e., in a way that was consistent with normal eating behavior). The mean values for the EDI-2 subscales under the honest condition were consistent with published norms, whereas the mean values for the faked condition were significantly different (and less indicative of disordered eating) from both the honest condition and published norms. Interestingly, the two subscales that are thought to be the most effective for identifying disordered eating and are used most frequently as screening tools (i.e., Drive for Thinness and Body Dissatisfaction) were the ones that differed most between the honest and the faked conditions. For example, in the honest condition, as would be expected, not one subject expressed complete satisfaction with the shape and size of her body (which would be represented by a score of zero on the Body Dissatisfaction subscale). However, in the faked condition, every subject scored a zero on the Body Dissatisfaction subscale.

The fake profile established in the first study was then used in a second study to screen 25 female collegiate gymnasts and 25 age-, height-, and weight-matched nonathletic controls for symptoms of disordered eating. Interestingly, 12% of the subjects had EDI-2 scores that matched the

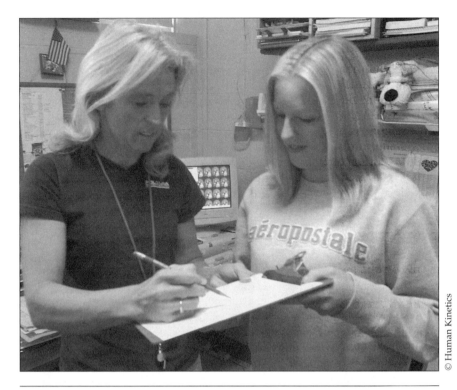

© Human Kinetics

There is currently no single fail-safe method or tool for identifying disordered eating in athletes. However, researchers and practitioners consider the personal interview to be one of the more accurate assessment tools.

empirically derived fake profile that was generated in the first study. These data and those from other studies by Wilmore (1991) highlight the limitations of self-report instruments and underscore the need for additional screening tools for accurate identification and assessment of disordered eating in athletes.

Interviews

Because of the limitations imposed by self-report screening instruments, many researchers and practitioners have suggested that interviewing athletes may be more accurate and therefore effective for identifying disordered eating behaviors. The study by Sundgot-Borgen (1993b) initially described in chapter 2 supports this recommendation. In this study a two-stage screening procedure was used to identify eating disorders in 522 elite Norwegian female athletes participating in 35 different sports. Athletes were initially screened for disordered eating using the EDI and were subsequently subjected to a clinical interview to verify the results of the EDI screen. When the data from the EDI were compared with those of the clinical interview, it was found that the EDI consistently underreported the prevalence of eating disorders as well as the frequency and severity of eating disorder symptoms and pathogenic weight control behaviors. The author concluded that interviews are absolutely essential for the accurate identification of disordered eating in athletes.

The increased accuracy afforded by the interview is likely due to a number of factors, all of which are related to the greater personal contact that an interview provides. A face-to-face interview allows direct contact between the interviewer and the interviewee. This establishes an immediate connection and fosters a degree of trust between the interviewer and interviewee, which makes it more difficult (and less desirable) for the interviewee to conceal behaviors, mask feelings or emotions, or lie. In addition, an interview provides for greater flexibility both in terms of the questions that can be asked and the responses that can be given. Generally, interviews consist of some if not all open-ended questions. These kinds of questions are advantageous in two ways. First, they give the interviewee greater flexibility in his or her responses (i.e., the respondent is not forced to select a response from a predetermined list). Second, open-ended questions provide the interviewer with an opportunity to probe and better interpret complex or ambiguous questions.

For example, a forced-response questionnaire might present the statement "I enjoy eating high-fat foods" and provide a Likert scale ranging from 1 (never) to 6 (always). This forces the respondent to choose between a limited number of predetermined frequencies. On the other hand, an interview question might ask if there are any foods that the respondent refuses to eat to examine food avoidance behaviors or ask for a description of food intake over the course of the week to ascertain regimented eating patterns. Finally, an in-depth interview allows the probing of issues that might require further clarification, something that cannot be achieved with a structured or forced-response questionnaire. Using the previous example question (*Are there any foods you avoid?*), if the interviewee had indicated an avoidance of high-fat foods, the interviewer could have probed further to find out why. Avoidance may be due to a fear that high-fat foods will cause weight gain, or it may be because high-fat foods cause the interviewee severe gastrointestinal distress (or the respondent suffers from hyperlipidemia and was told to avoid high-fat foods by a doctor).

The choice of conducting an individual (one-on-one with the athlete) or group (entire team) interview depends largely on the team dynamics. That is, a group interview is probably best suited for a close-knit team, one in which the athletes trust one another and feel secure that their revelations will be accepted and protected by the group. On the other hand, individual interviews are more appropriate for more individualized sports or teams in which the athletes are not as close or supportive, as individual interviews allow athletes to speak about their feelings without fear of censure from teammates. For example, an athlete may feel embarrassed about discussing his body image issues in front of teammates or may worry that they will ridicule him. Similarly, an athlete may fear that disclosing the details of her bulimic behaviors will elicit disgust or disdain from her teammates.

Regardless of the interview format (i.e., group or individual), the key to securing open and honest responses from the athletes lies in providing a safe, nonthreatening interview environment. Because athletes may feel intimidated by or fear the repercussions from coaches, trainers, and athletic administrators, it is probably best that the interview be conducted by an individual from outside the immediate athletic environment. Someone who has knowledge about and experience with disordered eating in athletes, such as a sport psychologist, sport dietitian, or team physician, is the most appropriate person to conduct the interview.

How the interview is conducted is just as important as who conducts the interview. The interview should be carried out in a manner that can ascertain the nature and extent of disordered eating behaviors without being judgmental or accusatory. Interview questions should assess eating behaviors, weight loss attempts, menstrual irregularities, and history of musculoskeletal injury (Johnson 1992; Nattiv et al. 1994; Otis et al. 1997). Other issues such as life stressors, depressive symptoms, dissatisfaction with weight or body shape, training frequency and intensity, and other lifestyle behaviors may provide additional pertinent information. A number of structured interviews for evaluating symptoms of disordered eating have been described in the literature, although only two—the Eating Disorder Examination (EDE; Cooper and Fairburn 1993; Fairburn and Cooper 1997) and the Interview for Diagnosis of Eating Disorders (IDED; Williamson 1990)—have been sufficiently tested and shown to be both valid and reliable. A description of these two instruments along with their strengths and limitations is presented in table 8.2.

Physiological Screening: The New Gold Standard?

Black et al. (in press) recently developed an eating disorder screening instrument that was shown to be superior to the EDI-2 and the BULIT-R in identifying female athletes with the full spectrum of disordered eating conditions. The Physiologic Screening Test (PST) is an 18-item instrument composed of 4 physical measurements—percentage body fat, waist-to-hip ratio, standing diastolic blood pressure, and parotid gland enlargement—and 14 self-report items assessing both physiological symptoms (e.g., dizziness, abdominal bloating and cramping not associated with menstrual periods, amenorrhea) and behaviors and cognitions (e.g., excessive exercise, body dissatisfaction, weight loss attempts) consistent with disordered eating. In a recent validation study, 148 female collegiate athletes were assessed using four eating disorder screening instruments: two commonly used eating disorder questionnaires normalized for the general population (EDI-2 and BULIT-R), the PST, and the Eating Disorder Examination (a validated, structured interview that was used for criterion validity). The PST was found to be more sensitive (i.e., the ability of the test to correctly identify those with disordered eating) and specific (i.e., the ability of the test to identify those without eating disorders) than both the EDI-2 and BULIT-R. In addition, the PST produced fewer false negatives and had greater negative predictive value, yield, accuracy, and validity than

Table 8.2 Structured Interviews for Identifying and Assessing Disordered Eating in Athletes

Instrument	Description	Strengths	Limitations
Eating Disorder Examination (EDE; Cooper and Fairburn 1987; Fairburn and Cooper 1993)	A semistructured interview for assessing symptoms associated with anorexia and bulimia nervosa that contains 4 subscales: (1) restraint, (2) eating concern, (3) shape concern, and (4) weight concern. The items derived from the interview are 23 symptom ratings made by the interviewer. The EDE has been updated or revised 12 times since its inception in 1987.	• Psychometric properties have been tested in many empirical studies • Inter-rater reliability of the individual symptom ratings and the subscale scores have been reported to be quite high • Has been used as a screening instrument in studies involving athletes	• No formal tests of its validity as a tool for diagnosing eating disorders have been conducted. • A qualified professional is required to conduct the interview and interpret the results. • It has not been formally validated in an athletic population.
Interview for Diagnosis of Eating Disorders, 4th ed. (IDED; Williamson 1990)	A semistructured interview for diagnosing anorexia nervosa, bulimia nervosa, and binge-eating disorder. DSM-IV criteria were used to structure the questions and develop the 21 symptom ratings. Diagnoses are based on high symptom ratings, which are the sum of the ratings for each symptom within each diagnostic category.	• Developed specifically for diagnosing eating disorders • Diagnosis of subtypes for anorexia and bulimia nervosa are operationalized • Inter-rater reliability and test–retest reliability have been reported to be high • Evidence for concurrent validity has been reported	• A qualified professional is required to conduct the interview and interpret the results. • It has not been validated in an athletic population.

either of the other two questionnaires. Finally, because the PST incorporates several *objective* physiological measures and can easily and unobtrusively be included as part of the preparticipation physical exam, its true purpose is more readily disguised, which may further minimize response bias and lead to even greater validity.

When to Screen for Disordered Eating

Just as important as which screening protocol (or protocols) to use is *when* to conduct the screening. The timing of eating disorder screening can have a significant impact on the validity of the results. The preparticipation physical exam is often considered the most opportune time to screen for disordered eating behaviors (Johnson 1992; Nattiv and Lynch 1994; Tanner 1994). Nonetheless, although convenient, the preparticipation physical may not provide the best setting for obtaining accurate information regarding disordered eating behaviors. Preparticipation physicals are frequently conducted en masse and thus are understandably quite hectic. There are typically three or four lengthy questionnaires to complete, and athletes are often in a hurry to get through them. Feeling somewhat overwhelmed and hurried, athletes are apt to respond hastily and haphazardly to questionnaires (particularly those assessing disordered eating behaviors). Moreover,

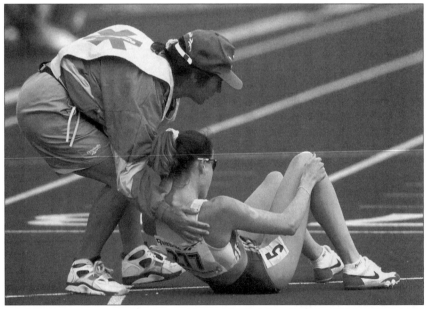

© Sport the Library

Observing behavior and performance can be the best way to identify disordered eating. Individuals who have daily contact with athletes (e.g., coaches, trainers, teammates) should possess a thorough knowledge of the signs and symptoms of disordered eating.

completing questionnaires in a group is likely to bias response due to peer pressure and the social desireability factor.

According to a recent study that assessed the athlete's view of the preparticipation physical exam (Carek and Futrell 1999), many athletes, particularly female athletes, feel uncomfortable discussing disordered eating during the preparticipation physical and thus may be apt to withhold information regarding their disordered eating behaviors. For these reasons it may be better (i.e., yield more accurate results) to conduct eating disorder screenings and interviews at another time, such as during the first few weeks of the season.

Direct Observation or Interaction

Sometimes simply observing the athlete's behavior is the best way to identify disordered eating (Ryan 1992a). Individuals who have daily contact with athletes (e.g., coaches, trainers, teammates) are in the best position to recognize behaviors that are consistent with disordered eating, such as excessive criticism of body weight, overly stringent eating patterns, refusal to eat with the team on road trips, and increased isolation from the team. Thus, it is essential that all those working closely with athletes as well as the athletes themselves possess a thorough knowledge of the signs and symptoms of disordered eating. Figure 8.1 lists some common warning signs

Behavioral
- Excessive criticism of one's body weight or shape
- Preoccupation with food, calories, or weight
- Compulsive, excessive exercise
- Mood swings, irritability
- Depression
- Social withdrawl
- Secretly eating or stealing food
- Bathroom visits after eating
- Avoiding food-related social activities
- Excessive use of laxatives, diuretics, or diet pills
- Consumption of large amounts of food inconsistent with the athlete's weight
- Excessive fear of being overweight or becoming fat that does not diminish as weight loss continues
- Preoccupation with the dietary patterns and eating behaviors of other people
- Lack of concern for excessive weight loss or extremely low body weight

Physical
- Chronic fatigue
- Noticeable weight loss or gain
- Anemia
- Frequent gastrointestinal problems or complaints (e.g., excessive gas, abdominal bloating, constipation, ulcers)
- Cold intolerance
- Lanugo (fine hair on the face and body)
- Tooth erosion, excessive dental caries
- Callused fingers
- Frequent musculoskeletal injuries (particularly stress fractures)
- Delayed or prolonged healing of wounds or injuries
- Frequent or prolonged illnesses
- Dry skin and hair
- Brittle nails
- Alopecia (hair loss)
- In women, irregular or absent menstrual cycles

Figure 8.1 Warning signs and symptoms of disordered eating in female athletes.

and symptoms of disordered eating in athletes. The National Collegiate
Athletic Association (NCAA) has also published a list of warning signs for
eating disorders that may be useful to coaches, athletes, and athletic staff
(www.ncaa.org).

Summary

The longer an eating disorder persists without treatment, the more severe
the consequences to the athlete's health and performance. Thus, early identification and subsequent intervention is essential to limiting the progression
and shortening the duration of disordered eating among athletes. While
a variety of eating disorder questionnaires and screening instruments are
available, none are without weaknesses limiting their validity and reliability. Thus, the best method for identifying athletes with disordered eating
is probably direct observation. For direct observation to be effective each
and every individual who works closely with athletes needs to be familiar
with the warning signs and symptoms of disordered eating.

nine

Treatment Considerations for Athletes With Disordered Eating

CHAPTER OBJECTIVES

After reading this chapter, you will be able to

- describe the history of eating disorder treatments;

- describe psychosocial treatment settings, including individual, family, and group therapies;

- discuss nutrition management as an integral part of eating disorder treatment;

- explain pharmacological options available for disordered eating;

- identify the benefits and risks associated with exercise as a form of adjunct therapy; and

- describe various experiential therapies, such as art, music, and dance or movement therapies.

The author wishes to thank Justine J. Reel, PhD, NCC, and Holly M. Estes, MS, University of Utah, for contributing this chapter.

Eating Disorder Treatment: Past and Present

The treatment of anorexia nervosa dates back to the late 1800s. Because little was known about the psychological underpinnings of anorexia nervosa at that time, early treatment focused on modifying the patient's eating behaviors rather than correcting the underlying psychological, cognitive, and affective components contributing to the eating disorder. The cornerstones of treatment were bed rest and a highly regimented diet, which included force-feeding of milk, cream, soup, eggs, fish, and chicken every two hours (Brumberg 1988; Gleaves et al. 2000). In addition, anorexic patients were routinely removed from their homes and isolated from family and friends. Treatment "success" was measured primarily by weight gain.

In the early 1900s physicians began to look at anorexia nervosa as more of a biologically based disease resulting from hormonal insufficiencies. Treatment regimens reflected this new line of thinking and anorexic patients were treated with a variety of substances thought to correct the hormonal imbalances, such as pituitary extract, insulin, estrogen, thyroid extract, and corticosteroids (Brumberg 1988; Parry-Jones 1985). It was not until the 1930s that medical professionals acknowledged the psychological aspects of anorexia nervosa and began to incorporate psychotherapy into the treatment regimen.

The treatment of bulimia does not share the rich past to that of anorexia largely because bulimia nervosa was much more recently delineated as a clinical eating disorder. Although bingeing and purging behaviors were observed during the early 1900s, bulimia nervosa was not defined as a specific eating disorder until 1979 (Russell 1979). As was true of anorexia nervosa, physicians historically focused on the disordered eating behaviors rather than on the underlying psychological issues that gave rise to these behaviors. Thus, treatment for bulimia nervosa centered on eliminating patients' voracious appetites by imposing regimented diets and prescribing various medicines that were supposed to warm the stomach (and theoretically create a feeling of fullness). As was true for anorexia nervosa, it wasn't until the mid-1900s that the focus of treatment shifted more toward the psychological aspects of bulimia nervosa. During this time psychologists worked to alleviate the hysteria and depressed mood that often plagued those with bulimia nervosa (Gleaves et al. 2000).

Treatment for eating disorders has come a long way since the early 1900s. Today treatments focus on both the underlying psychopathologies *and* the overt behaviors using a variety of modalities and protocols including individual, family, and group psychotherapy; nutritional counseling; medications; and, more recently, experiential therapies (art, music, and movement) and exercise therapy. Most importantly, today's treatments are individualized, tailored to best meet the needs of each individual patient. This is particularly important for the athlete with disordered eating who often has issues that are unique to the athletic setting.

This chapter describes the various types of eating disorder treatments currently available, including psychosocial, nutrition management, pharmacological, exercise, and experiential therapies. Those treatment modalities that may be particularly relevant or effective for athletes are highlighted. The goal of the chapter is to provide health professionals with a deeper understanding of treatment modalities so that they can help their athletes make informed treatment decisions. It should be emphasized that the role of dietitians, coaches, athletic trainers, and other health professionals is to connect athletes suspected of having disordered eating with specialized treatment for eating disorders rather than actually implementing treatment themselves.

Types of Eating Disorder Treatments and Their Relevance for Athletes

As was shown in chapters 1 and 3, athletes with disordered eating demonstrate subtle but significant differences in eating disorder symptoms and etiology from their nonathletic counterparts. Thus, optimal treatment for athletes should address the aspects of disordered eating that are unique to athletes. For example, treatment for nonathletes who demonstrate compulsive exercise behaviors generally involves restricting physical activity in order to reduce the dependence on exercise. This line of treatment would be not only difficult but also probably counterproductive for the athlete who must continue to train to be competitive in his or her sport.

Ideally, the treatment of eating disorders in athletes should include a variety of modalities, including psychosocial interventions, nutritional management, and in certain circumstances pharmacological interventions. Exercise and experiential therapies have also been prescribed as potential adjunct treatment modalities for disordered eating. This section describes the currently available treatment modalities for disordered eating and their pertinence to athletes.

Psychosocial Interventions

Psychological counseling is the cornerstone of treatment for disordered eating for both athletes and nonathletes. A variety of psychological approaches have been used successfully in both populations, including psychodynamic, behavioral, and cognitive-behavioral approaches. Psychodynamic approaches focus on the roles of childhood experiences, attachment issues, and relationship dynamics (e.g., mother–daughter bond) in the development and maintenance of the disordered eating behaviors. Behavioral approaches emphasize identifying environmental cues that precipitate or trigger the disordered eating behaviors and then attempting to reduce those cues (e.g., stimulus control). For example, a behavioral therapist might ask a bulimic patient to identify triggers (e.g., stress, critical remarks) that precipitate the binge–purge cycle and then help him or her formulate a new healthy response as an alternative to bingeing and purging (Goodsitt 1997; Polivy and Federoff 1997). Highly regarded cognitive-behavioral approaches involve identifying dysfunctional thought patterns (e.g., "I am a bad person") that trigger disordered eating behaviors (Stein et al.

2001) and then reshaping those thought patterns to reduce the disordered eating behaviors.

The challenge of eating disorder treatment is that in most cases therapy is largely involuntary; that is, the patient is often a reluctant participant. Therefore, finding the therapeutic approach that most closely fits the needs of the patient with disordered eating is a critical aspect of the recovery process. Variables to consider when determining a treatment approach include the treatment setting (e.g., inpatient vs. outpatient) and format (e.g., individual vs. group, with or without family).

Treatment Setting

The treatment of disordered eating can be conducted in an inpatient or outpatient setting (or both). In most cases, the severity and chronicity of the disordered eating behaviors dictates whether treatment will be conducted on an inpatient or outpatient basis, although other factors may ultimately influence the decision (e.g., suicidal tendencies, co-morbid conditions, unsafe family environment).

Inpatient Treatment   Hospitalization or treatment at a residential care facility that specializes in eating disorders is generally reserved for those eating disorder patients whose physical or psychological health is in immediate jeopardy. Kaplan and Sadock (1998) suggested that anorexic individuals who are 20% below their expected weight for height be treated on an inpatient basis. Inpatient treatment should also be provided if the patient with disordered eating demonstrates suicidal tendencies, appears to be at risk of self-destructive behaviors (e.g., self-mutilation) or suffers debilitating depression (Thompson and Sherman 1993). The length of the inpatient treatment is largely determined by the amount of weight lost and the severity of accompanying medical complications. Kaplan and Sadock (1998) indicated that a patient who is 30% below expected weight could likely remain hospitalized for two to six months.

The advantages of treatment in an inpatient setting are that it provides a structured environment in which the patient has access to clinical support and health care professionals can monitor the eating disorder patient around the clock. The disadvantages of inpatient treatment are that it can be quite costly, treatment can be lengthy, and relapse is likely, especially if the treatment facility lacks a re-integration plan for helping the patient re-enter the real world. Residential care facilities (e.g., Center for Change, Renfrew Hospitals) provide an alternative to inpatient treatment in the general hospital setting; however, these treatment facilities are not always easily accessible to individuals in rural communities or to individuals with limited health insurance plans. In fact, most insurance plans do not cover extended visits beyond stabilization of patients.

Because of the scarcity of inpatient treatment facilities, it is not uncommon for eating disorder patients to have to travel some distance to seek specialized treatment. In this case local hospitals will typically fulfill the eating disordered patients' immediate medical needs, stabilize them, and then send them on to an inpatient or outpatient program specializing in the treatment of eating disorders.

Outpatient Treatment   Outpatient treatment is considered appropriate when the patient with disordered eating is not in immediate medical jeopardy (e.g., no immediate medical dangers, no significant psychological co-morbidities, body weight is stable and not exceedingly low). Outpatient treatment is similar to inpatient treatment (in terms of therapeutic components) except that the patient does not reside at the facility where he or she is being treated. Instead, the patient generally comes into the facility for treatment 1-3 times per week (depending upon his or her needs). Historically, bulimic patients have been treated on an outpatient basis more often than those with anorexia nervosa (Thompson and Sherman 1993).

The advantages of outpatient treatment facilities are that they tend to be less costly than inpatient facilities and, by allowing patients to remain in their normal or regular environments they may reduce the risk of relapse. That is, since patients in the outpatient setting have not been removed completely from the real world, they may be better able to adapt to life in the real world after treatment. On the other hand, returning to their regular environment between treatments could be disastrous for some patients since the factors contributing to development and maintenance of their disorder may be their home environment.

An option for those eating disorder patients needing more structure than what the typical outpatient facility provides is a form of partial psychiatric hospitalization known as Intensive Outpatient Therapy (IOP). More intense than weekly outpatient therapy but less intense than inpatient hospitalization, IOP involves a range of therapeutic modalities several days per week for several hours at a time.

Although outpatient programs or psychotherapists can usually be found in the Yellow Pages of the phone book, it may be helpful for health professionals to obtain a list of referrals and background information on possible programs and practitioners specializing in the treatment of athletes with disordered eating. Health professionals can call eating disorder specialists to ascertain their credentials, years of experience, and references. Psychotherapists may be either master's level or doctoral clinicians in an array of helping professions: clinical social work (MSW), clinical or counseling psychology (PhD or PsyD), counselor education (LPC), psychiatry (MD), or psychiatric nursing (RN). The clinician's degree is less important than formal training in and experience with treating disordered eating.

To aid practitioners in determining the most appropriate treatment setting for a given eating disorder patient, the American Psychiatric Association (1999) established the following set of guidelines or levels of care:

- Level 1 (outpatient treatment)
- Level 2 (intensive outpatient treatment)
- Level 3 (partial hospitalization)

- Level 4 (residential health care facility)
- Level 5 (inpatient hospitalization)

The level of care the patient receives is generally based on the following factors: medical complications, suicidal tendencies, body weight, motivation to recover, environmental stress, purging behavior, other disorders present, treatment availability, and structure needed for eating and gaining weight. Thus, level 1 treatment would be appropriate for patients who are medically stable, have no suicidal ideations, have good motivation to recover, and are self-sufficient. In contrast, level 5 care would be best suited for patients with severe medical conditions (e.g., electrolyte imbalances, extremely low body weight), suicidal intent, or other psychiatric disorders and who likely require intravenous fluids or feedings (Muscari 2002).

Treatment Format

Individuals with disordered eating can receive psychological counseling on an individual basis or in a group setting or both. Similarly, they can be counseled with or without family members present. There are advantages and disadvantages to each format, and for this reason a variety of formats often are used during different phases of treatment. The format chosen should be specific to the patient's individual needs and underlying core issues, regardless of athletic participation. The various treatment formats are described in the following paragraphs.

Individual Therapy   Individual therapy involves the patient meeting one-on-one with a therapist. Although eating behaviors are often discussed, the surrounding emotional issues are the primary focus of therapy sessions. The specific issues covered will vary somewhat, depending on the therapist's theoretical orientation (e.g., cognitive-behavioral, psychodynamic) and the patient's needs. The advantages of individual therapy are that the athlete receives undivided attention and has the opportunity to probe in-depth into personal issues that have contributed to disordered eating (Thompson and Sherman 1993). A disadvantage is that individual therapy does not address family interaction variables and the impact that they may have had on the etiology and maintenance of the disordered eating behaviors.

Family Therapy   Boskind-White and White (1991) tied disordered eating to surrounding family conditions and argued that the family system creates and enables unhealthful behaviors. Thus, a key benefit of family therapy is the ability to gain insight into the role that the athlete plays within his or her family. Indeed, according to Nichols and Schwartz (1995, p. 69), "Once therapists began to view people in the context of the family, their behavior not only seemed less strange, but it could be understood as an inevitable and necessary aspect of the way the family has evolved." The ideal aims of family therapy are to change the factors within the family system that are causing the patient distress and to facilitate communication between the patient and family. Family therapy intends to create a supportive family system rather

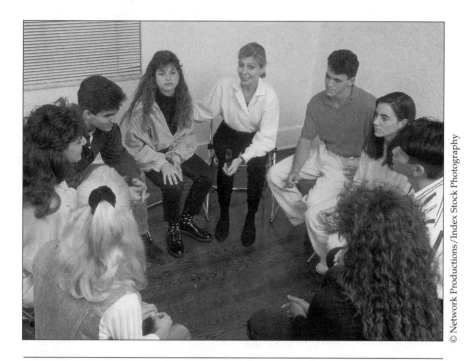

Group therapy is advantageous for athletes because it provides a team environment.

than blaming family culprits (Lackstrom and Woodside 1998). Assessing the family dynamics is an integral part of understanding interactions that perpetuate the disorder (American Psychiatric Association 2000).

The few controlled family therapy studies have used the Maudsley approach, which entails three phases for family therapy and encompasses 15 sessions over a period of 8 to 14 months. During the first phase, a family effort is made to help the patient resume normal eating. Once the patient has gained sufficient body weight, the focus shifts to family issues unrelated to eating. In the final stage of therapy, the sessions focus on defining appropriate family roles and setting boundaries (Stein et al. 2001).

Group Therapy   Group therapy usually involves forming a treatment group of other individuals with disordered eating. The group format allows self-disclosure, catharsis, and insight. In addition, disordered eating is often a private disorder, so the group allows "public" disclosure in a safe environment, an important step toward recovery (Hobbs et al. 1989). The goal of group treatment is to help a client identify feelings, needs, wishes, and goals. "By listening to other members, patients begin to pay attention to their inner experience and learn to identify, to own, and to articulate their feelings" (Baumann 1992, p. 96).

Athletes may especially appreciate the camaraderie of a group, which can share some of the social benefits of belonging to a team. It is highly unlikely that all members of an eating disorder group will be athletes, but by interacting with other individuals who are struggling with similar issues, the athlete with disordered eating is able to avoid social isolation, a common characteristic among individuals with anorexia and bulimia nervosa. Socialization skills can be practiced in the group setting, and the athlete is able to interact with individuals beyond his or her family and team (Thompson and Sherman 1993). A group setting is ideal for clients with disordered eating to share common experiences and to educate and provide support for one another (Costin 1999).

Nutritional Management

Nutritional counseling, ideally provided by a registered dietitian, is considered a key component in the total treatment regimen for disordered eating. While psychotherapy aims to uncover and correct the underlying psychological issues fueling the disordered eating, nutritional counseling focuses on changing the overt behaviors, that is, the disordered eating itself. The goal of nutritional counseling is to re-educate the patient and reintroduce and reinforce normal eating behaviors.

Individuals suffering from disordered eating often appear to be "experts" in nutrition. Many eating disorder patients can readily recite the calorie content of foods (particularly forbidden foods), often better than most registered dietitians. However, individuals with eating disorders generally lack a true understanding of nutritional concepts; the nutrition "knowledge" they do possess tends to be highly distorted, fraught with myths and misconceptions. Moreover, individuals with eating disorders have often been locked in abnormal eating patterns for so long that they have no concept of what constitutes normal or healthful eating. Thus, the primary goals of nutritional management are to dispel the myths and misconceptions regarding food and diet and to reestablish healthful eating patterns. The specific objectives of nutritional therapy are similar for both anorexic and bulimic patients and include allaying the fears associated with food and eating, learning to recognize and respond to feelings of hunger and satiety, and establishing healthful eating behaviors.

As was described in depth in chapter 1, both anorexics and bulimics are terrified of food. They fear losing control around food and the potential consequences of that loss of control (i.e., weight gain). Nutritional counseling therefore should center on helping the patient with an eating disorder overcome his or her food phobias. One approach is to replace fear with facts. That is, providing accurate information on such topics as energy balance, vitamin and mineral functions and requirements, and fluid needs may help to ease food anxieties. In addition, meal management (i.e., creating meal plans and strategies to deal with irrational food thoughts and behaviors) can aid in reducing the fear associated with eating and can also be used to empower the patient to take control of mealtimes and food intake. For example, an anorexic patient who follows his or her eating plan may receive positive reinforcement for food consumed or weight gained in the form of increased independence (Martin 1998).

Most patients with disordered eating have completely lost touch with internal (physiological) feelings of hunger and satiety and instead rely on external cues and rigid rules for eating. For anorexics, denying hunger and adhering to strict dietary rules becomes the cornerstone of their disorder. Similarly, bulimics learn to override satiety while engaging in binge eating behavior. Thus, nutritional counseling must focus on helping patients recognize and respond appropriately to bodily signals of hunger and satiety (Kahm 2001). One of the most effective tools for reestablishing the physiological sense of hunger and satiety is the food log. Recording not only what they eat, but when, why (in response to what internal or external cues), and where they eat increases the patients' awareness and allows the appropriate manipulation of external cues to produce the desired behavior (referred to by behaviorists as *stimulus control*). For example, many anorexic individuals restrict their energy intake to less than 800 kcal/d and avoid fat, sugar, or both. Using a food log, the dietitian can clearly illustrate the nutritional inadequacy of this diet and then reeducate the patient about normal-sized food portions by showing food models (Garfinkel 1996). Similarly, the bulimic patient can use the food log to gain a better understanding of the factors (e.g., thoughts, feelings, situations) that precipitate a binge and use this information to reduce environmental and emotional triggers in the future. Food logs can also be used to monitor changes in the patient's eating behaviors. Progress and lapses become tangible because there is a physical record of the patient's eating behaviors.

The specific outcomes of nutritional therapy differ somewhat for anorexic and bulimic patients. For the bulimic patient, the primary nutritional objective is to reduce bingeing and purging behaviors (APA 2000). The primary nutritional outcome for the anorexic patient, on the other hand, is to restore and maintain a healthy body weight (Muscari 2002). Caution should be taken when instituting weight gain in anorexic patients. Refeeding syndrome or extremely rapid weight gain can lead to cardiac problems (e.g., congestive heart failure). Typical treatment involves gaining no more than 2 lb (0.9 kg) per week.

Pharmacological Treatment

Psychotropic medications (i.e., medications used to treat mood disorders such as antidepressants) are sometimes included in the eating disorder treatment regimen. It should be emphasized that these medications are used to treat the *symptoms* that accompany disordered eating (e.g., anxiety, depression) as opposed to treating the eating disorder itself. Generally speaking, medications tend to be more routinely prescribed for those with bulimia nervosa than anorexia nervosa. Because medications may be used as an adjunct treatment to traditional counseling, health professionals should have knowledge of which medications are most commonly prescribed and their effectiveness and potential side effects.

Antidepressants have been shown to be effective for treating the mood disorders that often afflict individuals with bulimia nervosa. For example, Hudson, Pope, and Carter (1999) reported that antidepressants helped to reduce bulimic patients' preoccupation with food and weight. In addition, their clinical trials showed that antidepressants promoted a decrease in patients' bingeing and vomiting episodes. Similarly, Martin (1998) reported a decrease in bingeing by 50% in the majority of eating disordered patients being treated with antidepressants. Elizabeth Joy, a team physician at the University of Utah who routinely treats athletes with eating disorders (see chapter 11), reported that she has had success with antidepressant medications, particularly in her bulimic patients. In a recent article (Sample 2000) Dr. Joy indicated that 75% of her eating disorder clients are using antidepressant therapy. According to Joy, Prozac has helped to reduce purging behaviors in some bulimic patients, theoretically by elevating their serotonin levels.

Unfortunately, despite research supporting the efficacy of antidepressants for treating bulimia nervosa, their effectiveness in treating anorexia nervosa remains questionable (Kaye 1999). For example, Wilson and Agras (2001) indicated that antidepressant medications are inefficacious in treating acutely underweight, malnourished, anorexic patients. Moreover, anorexics may be more susceptible to adverse side effects. Nevertheless, Wilson and Agras (2001) recanted somewhat by suggesting that antidepressants may be effective in preventing relapse and treating underlying mood disorders among weight-restored anorexic clients.

Muscari (2002) attempted to identify alternative medications to antidepressants to expand the treatment efficacy of medication and reported that low-dose neuroleptic drugs can be prescribed to decrease anxiety, severe obsessive thoughts, and psychosis. Case reports have demonstrated the efficacy of olanzapine (a neuroleptic typically prescribed for schizophrenia) for improving weight gain and maintenance and reducing anxiety in anorexic clients in an inpatient setting (Boachie, Goldfield, and Spettigue 2003).

Other medications, such as mood stabilizers (e.g., lithium carbonate), have been used sporadically for treatment of bulimic patients. These medications appear to be most useful for the treatment of bulimic patients who also suffer from bipolar affective disorder (Hudson, Pope, and Carter 1999). Appetite stimulants, such as clonidine, have demonstrated some limited success in weight restoration in anorexic patients (Kaye 1999).

Psychotropic medications are typically prescribed by a physician, psychiatrist, or, in some states (e.g., New Mexico), a clinical psychologist. It should be emphasized that pharmacological interventions alone cannot treat eating disorders among athletes, and thus they should not be the sole form of treatment. Nonetheless, certain psychotropic medications can help alleviate symptoms associated with disordered eating and thus are a helpful dimension of the total treatment plan.

A concern expressed by many athletes, coaches, and trainers is what effect psychotropic medications have on athletic performance. It is a legitimate concern as the drugs used in treating disordered eating are not without side effects that could potentially negatively affect athletic performance. For example, antidepressant drugs may cause diaphoresis (i.e., excessive sweating), gastrointestinal distress, nausea, drowsiness, and dizziness (Lacy et al. 2002), all of which could impair athletic performance. Nonetheless, in some cases the benefits of taking the medication may outweigh the possible side effects. For example, psychotropic medications can reduce psychological symptoms (e.g., depression, anxiety) that impede athletic training and may also increase self-confidence and enthusiasm for the sport (Schwenk 1997; Otis and Goldingay 2000; Lacy et al. 2002) thereby indirectly enhancing athletic performance. The prescribing physician should closely monitor the athlete initially for adverse reactions to the medication and adjust treatment accordingly.

Certain side effects can be managed to allow the athlete to continue sport participation. For example, if the athlete experiences an increase in sweating, he or she can adjust fluid intake to cover the additional fluid loss. If drowsiness occurs, the athlete may need to modify the dose or alter the timing of the mediation (i.e., take two smaller doses per day or take the medication at night before going to bed). The likelihood of side effects may be decreased by using lower dosages of the medication at first and then gradually increasing the dosage if necessary (Joy et al. 1997b; Zetin and Tate 1999). If the patient suffers excruciating side effects, the physician may prescribe a different medication, or stop the medication entirely.

Exercise Therapy

Using exercise as a treatment modality for disordered eating is understandably controversial given the central role of exercise in the pathology of both anorexia and bulimia nervosa. That is, individuals with bulimia nervosa frequently use exercise as a purging method, while those with anorexia nervosa often engage in excessive exercise to maintain a significant negative energy balance and thus a low body weight. Moreover, athletes with disordered eating are already exercising at levels that most would consider excessive. Thus, it may seem counterintuitive (and even contraindicated) to prescribe exercise as a treatment for disordered eating, particularly in athletes. Lack of logic notwithstanding, recent research suggests that exercise may be beneficial as an adjunct form of treatment for individuals, including athletes, with disordered eating (Beumont et al. 1994). For example, physical activity could help empower clients to feel a sense of control over their own bodies in an otherwise restrictive environment. Similarly, exercise may be a strategy for minimizing the anxiety associated with weight gain in recovery. Rosenblum and Forman (2002, p. 381) argued that exercise "is a component of promoting healthy living, and it may be a motivating factor for some clients undergoing treatment." For athletes, permitting a minimal amount of exercise as part of the overall treatment plan allows them to hold on to a significant part of their self-concept (see chapters 1 and 3).

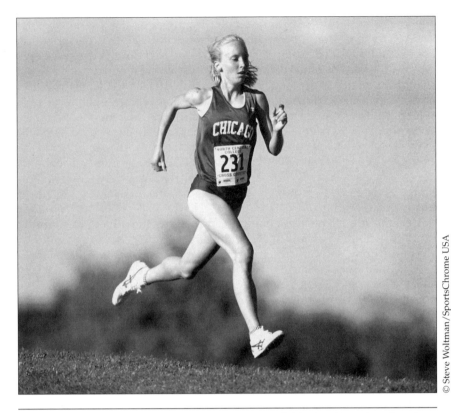

Exercise could be a viable form of treatment for individuals with eating disorders. Researchers have found that physical exercise can help to alleviate disordered eating characteristics (e.g., body dissatisfaction) more than nutritional counseling and cognitive-behavioral therapy.

Blinder, Freeman, and Stunkard (1970) discovered that while eating disorder patients attempted to conceal restrictive eating, they appeared to be more open about physical activity behaviors. In fact, therapists were able to use access to physical activity as a reward for patients who gained weight. "The coupling of a result of eating (weight gain) with an event reinforcing for the client (access to physical activity) permitted a therapeutic confrontation over relatively conflict-free behaviors to substitute for the traditional confrontation over the conflict-ridden behavior of eating" (Blinder, Freeman, and Stunkard 1970, p. 1098).

In a recent study, Sundgot-Borgen and colleagues (2002) compared nutritional counseling, cognitive-behavioral therapy, and physical exercise for the treatment of bulimia nervosa. The moderate-intensity exercise regimen consisted of a single one-hour group session per week and lasted for 16 weeks. The exercise regimen alleviated disordered eating characteristics (e.g., body dissatisfaction) more than the other modes of treatment, demonstrating that exercise could be a viable form of treatment for eating disorders.

Thien and colleagues (2000) has recommended a graded exercise protocol for disordered eating patients that varies based on the individual's body weight and percentage of body fat (table 9.1). The program includes seven levels through which a patient could move as treatment progressed. For example, level 1 includes stretching exercises three times a week in sitting and lying positions. Progressing to level 7 allows the addition of both strength and cardiovascular exercise (Thien et al. 2000).

Table 9.1   The Seven Levels of Exercise

Level	Patient's body composition	Exercise
1	<75% IBW or <19% BF	Stretching exercises 3×/wk, sitting and lying
2	75% IBW or 19% BF	Stretching exercises 3×/wk, stretching, sitting, and lying
3a	80% IBW or 20% BF	Stretching exercises 3×/wk; isometric exercise, 1 set 3×/wk for 3 wk
3b	80% IBW or 20% BF	Stretching exercises 3×/wk; isometric exercise, 2 sets 3×/wk; low-impact cardiovascular exercise, 2×/wk after 3 wk
4	85% IBW or 21% BF	Stretching exercises 3×/wk; isometric exercise 3×/wk; low-impact cardiovascular exercise 3×/wk
5	90% IBW or 22.5% BF	Stretching exercises 3×/wk; resistive strengthening, 1 set 3×/wk; low-impact cardiovascular exercise 3×/wk
6	95% IBW or 23.7% BF	Stretching exercises 3×/wk; resistive strengthening, 2 sets 3×/wk; low-impact cardiovascular exercise 3×/wk
7	100% IBW or 25% BF	Stretching exercises 3×/wk; resistive strengthening, 2-3 sets 3×/wk; low-impact cardiovascular exercise 3×/wk

The seven levels are described by Thien et al. (2000) and involve a gradual progression of activity level for eating disorder patients. The level is based on the patient's ideal body weight (IBW) and percentage of body fat (BF). All patients should begin at level 1 despite their IBW or BF and continue at each level for at least one week.

The Controversy of Exercise Therapy

Exercise is understandably a controversial form of treatment. However, the following rationales for using exercise as part of the eating disorder treatment have been put forward by Beumont and colleagues (1994): (1) it is time-consuming and challenging to attempt to police exercise behavior that is forbidden, (2) it is advantageous to educate clients about beneficial forms of exercise, and (3) exercise can provide a vehicle for client independence beyond the psychiatric unit. The following table describes some of the benefits of exercise for patients with eating disorders.

Benefits of Exercise Components for Eating Disorder Patients

Exercise component	Benefits
Flexibility	Reduces muscle tension, uses little energy, improves posture
Strength training	Restores lean body tissue,[*] increases body awareness
Social sport	Promotes teamwork and social interaction
Aerobic exercise[**]	Eases resumption of athletic training, educates about healthy amounts of exercise

[*] This assumes that the athlete is in a positive energy balance.

[**] Aerobic exercise should be low impact. Running is discouraged because it increases risk of orthopedic injury.

Despite the apparent benefits of exercise as a treatment for disordered eating, many practitioners and researchers remain skeptical. Many still feel the potential pitfalls of exercise outweigh any benefits. Indeed, there is a risk that the athlete will develop rigid rules for physical activity that will become another ritual of an obsessive-compulsive disorder. In addition, the athlete may be at risk for overtraining, injury, or more serious medical problems. Thus, until more definitive data become available, exercise should be prescribed with caution.

Experiential Therapies

In recent years, experiential therapies have become increasingly more common. Experiential therapies involve activities, such as art, music, dance or movement, and even horseback riding, that enable eating disorder patients to identify and express their feelings, sensations, and perceptions in a creative rather than a destructive manner (Hornyak and Baker 1989).

Experiential therapies provide an alternative approach to psychotherapy when an eating disorder patient is unable to verbalize his or her feelings and experiences within counseling sessions (Morenoff and Sobol 1989).

For example, art therapy allows individuals to display their perceptions about themselves, their environment, and their role within their surroundings through drawings or paintings (Morenoff and Sobol 1989). These images can then be used for discussion in psychotherapy sessions, which may help increase the productiveness and effectiveness of each meeting. Music therapy may be employed to help patients convey their emotions through singing, composition of lyrics, and musical sounds. Besides self-expression through music, listening to music may help the patient use stress-reduction strategies, such as deep breathing to a slow, peaceful tune, and may stimulate relevant thoughts, depending on the tempo, volume, and other characteristics of the music (Parente 1989).

Dance or movement therapy may be another useful experiential treatment modality. Dance therapies lead patients through activities that allow body exploration. Clients develop sensory awareness by identifying body signals, such as tension, pressure, or temperature; gain a more accurate understanding of how their bodies function; discover reasons to trust their bodies to function properly and perform certain actions; and express feelings through movement (Rice, Hardenbergh, and Hornyak 1989; Stark, Aronow, and McGeehan 1989).

Patients will most likely demonstrate a preference for the type of experiential therapy that is the most meaningful for them; however, experiential approaches are not as accessible as traditional psychotherapy. If available, experiential therapies provide a useful supplement to a larger eating disorder treatment program.

Summary

This chapter provided an overview of the various therapeutic approaches currently used to treat eating disorders in both athletic and non-athletic populations. Ideally treatment should include a combination of modalities including psychotherapy, nutritional counseling, medication, and possibly exercise and experiential therapies. Psychotherapy aims at uncovering and treating the underlying psychological issues related to the disordered eating behaviors and may include individual, family, or group approaches. Nutritional counseling is designed to dispel the myths and misconceptions surrounding diet and reinforce more healthful eating behaviors. Medication has been shown to be helpful as an adjunct treatment for the mood disorders and symptomatology related to the eating disorder. Exercise therapy, while still somewhat controversial, has been shown to be effective in reducing stress and improving the body image of eating disordered patients. Finally, experiential approaches such as dance, art, and music therapy have shown some promise, particularly for those being treated in inpatient facilities as they allow another outlet of expression.

Health professionals and athletic staff should realize that treatment of patients with disordered eating, including athletes, is a lengthy and complex process. Unlike a sport injury, disordered eating may prevent the athlete from sport participation even after medical signs of distress are absent. The recovery process is highly variable.

ten

Management of Athletes With Disordered Eating

CHAPTER OBJECTIVES

After reading this chapter, you will be able to

- identify the best way to approach an athlete with disordered eating,

- discuss referral guidelines,

- understand the options available when an athlete refuses treatment, and

- identify competition and participation issues related to eating disorders.

The author wishes to thank Justine J. Reel, PhD, NCC, and Holly M. Estes, MS University of Utah, for their contributions to this chapter.

Management Versus Treatment of Disordered Eating in Athletes

Management of disordered eating can be distinguished from treatment in a number of ways, including the procedures, time frame, and providers involved. As described in chapter 9, treatment of disordered eating involves the application of specific therapeutic modalities—psychological, nutritional, and medical—that commence *after* the eating disorder has been identified and continue just until it has resolved. Management, on the other hand, encompasses a broader range of measures conducted over a longer period of time, beginning with identification, including treatment, and continuing on through the posttreatment follow-up period (Thompson and Sherman 1993). Moreover, while only qualified health professionals are involved in treatment, managing disordered eating involves the cooperative efforts of not only health professionals but all those associated with the athlete, including coaches, trainers, parents, and sometimes even teammates.

This chapter describes the general guidelines for managing disordered eating in athletes. Specific strategies are presented delineating how to approach the athlete with disordered eating, provide referrals, and arrange for and monitor treatment and posttreatment care. Two case studies are included to aid in the understanding and application of the management guidelines presented.

Case Study 1: Cassie

Cassie was a 17-year-old high school cheerleader and amateur gymnast who was determined to cheer at the college level. At 5 ft 7 in. and 145 lb (170 cm and 65.8 kg), Cassie exceeded the university squad tryout weight limit for women (100-120 lb, or 45.4-54.4 kg). In an attempt to shed weight, Cassie began to exercise excessively, running seven days a week for at least an hour in addition to her cheerleading and gymnastics practice. Her daily energy intake rarely exceeded 600 kcal/d and consisted of mostly fruits, vegetables, and an occasional bagel. To speed up her weight loss process, Cassie began taking large doses of laxatives and diuretics. Within three months Cassie's weight dropped to 112 lb (50.8 kg), and she ceased to menstruate. Despite her weight loss, Cassie continued to view herself as grossly overweight. Cassie's private gymnastics instructor seemed pleased with her weight loss and complimented Cassie on her self-control and leaner shape. In contrast, Cassie's cheerleading coach grew concerned with her weight loss, excessive exercise, and increasingly derogatory remarks about her body weight and shape. While the cheerleading coach wanted to confront Cassie, she felt uncomfortable crossing personal boundaries with her athletes, so she just let it go.

Case Study 2: Michael

Michael, a collegiate wrestler, wrestled at two weight classes below his normal weight. In order to cut weight, he practiced various purging and dehydration strategies, including self-induced vomiting, spitting into a cup, running in a rubber suit, and sitting for hours in a sauna. While several of Michael's teammates also engaged in some of these pathogenic weight loss behaviors, none did so as frequently as Michael. Moreover, unlike his teammates, who practiced pathogenic weight control behaviors only during the season, Michael found that his purging behaviors persisted into the off-season. Michael became caught up in a vicious cycle of consuming large portions of food (up to 20,000 kcal in one sitting) and then trying to get rid of the food by vomiting or excessive exercise. Michael justified his purging behaviors by convincing himself that he was maintaining his competitive discipline off-season. However, deep inside, Michael felt out of control. Occasionally, Michael would wonder whether he should consider getting help, but he would end up convincing himself that only women are susceptible to eating disorders. He was just doing what he had to do to be a good wrestler. One of Michael's teammates confronted him about his eating disorder, accusing him of purging and threatening to expose him if he didn't get help. Needless to say, Michael felt betrayed and trapped; he denied the accusations vehemently and secretly vowed to be more careful and guarded about his purging behaviors in the future.

Steps for Managing Disordered Eating in Athletes

Management of disordered eating encompasses a sequential series of steps, including (1) approaching the athlete and convincing him or her to seek treatment; (2) providing referrals for treatment programs, facilities, or providers; (3) arranging for treatment; and (4) monitoring the athlete's progress during treatment and posttreatment follow-up to ensure the maintenance of therapeutic gains (Thompson and Sherman 1993). Each of these steps are described in the following sections; the case studies are referred to for ease of interpretation and application.

Approaching the Athlete with Disordered Eating

Approaching an athlete with disordered eating and convincing him or her to seek treatment can be an extremely difficult undertaking. Although the athlete with disordered eating may appear to be the most compliant person on the team, when threatened with exposure and the potential consequences (e.g., embarrassment, disapproval by coaches and teammates, being withheld from competition or removed from the team, having to relinquish the pathogenic weight control behaviors and possibly gain weight), denial and defiance often take over. Thus, it is crucial to be sensitive yet firm when approaching an athlete who is suspected of having an eating disorder and attempting to convince him or her to seek treatment. The potential for a successful intervention increases if the following three conditions are met: (1) the athlete is approached in a timely fashion, (2)

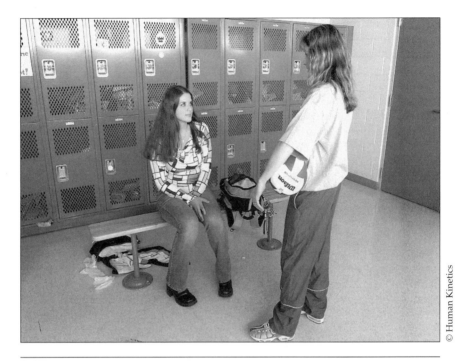

© Human Kinetics

When it comes to the treatment of eating disorders, it is crucial that the athlete be approached and persuaded to seek treatment as soon as possible after the disordered eating is identified.

there is an established rapport between the athlete and the individual attempting the intervention, and (3) the athlete is approached with caring and concern.

As was described in the previous chapter, when it comes to the treatment of eating disorders, time is truly of the essence. Because of the potentially serious medical consequences associated it is essential that athletes suffering from disordered eating begin treatment as soon as possible. Furthermore, researchers suggest that the longer the disorder is allowed to persist without treatment, the greater the recovery time (Hall and Ostroff 1999). Thus, it is crucial that the athlete be approached and persuaded to seek treatment as soon as possible after the disordered eating is identified.

Most practitioners agree that the best person to approach the athlete with an eating disorder is the one who has the best rapport with him or her *and* is in a position of authority (Thompson and Sherman 1993). While a teammate or friend may have the closest relationship with the athlete suffering from disordered eating, neither would be considered the best choice because they lack the authority, responsibility, resources, and experience necessary to provide the appropriate support during treatment and follow-up. The failed intervention attempt by Michael's teammate is a perfect example of why teammates should not be the ones to approach the athlete with disordered eating. Instead, it is generally recommended that a coach, assistant coach, athletic trainer, or counselor be the one to initially approach the eating disordered athlete.

Of equal if not greater importance to *who* approaches the athlete with an eating disorder is *how* the athlete is approached. Confronting the athlete in an accusing or reproachful manner is the worst approach, as it will likely lead to denial, anger, and defiance. Instead, the athlete should be approached with sincerity, respect, caring, and concern. In addition, it has been suggested that the emphasis not be placed on the specific disordered eating behaviors per se, but rather on the consequences of those behaviors (Ryan 1992a). For example, rather than point out that the athlete is eating only 500 kcal/d and exercising excessively, express concern for his or her decline in performance, depressed or erratic moods, obvious fatigue, frequent injuries, and so on. Michael's teammate would have undoubtedly been more successful if he had expressed concern for Michael's health and performance rather than hurling accusations and confronting him directly about his disordered eating behaviors. Research suggests that individuals with eating disorders are more likely to seek help for the resulting health problems than the disordered eating behaviors themselves (Holliman 1991).

Ohio State University's athletic department issued an eating disorder policy in 2001 (Hill 2001) with the following suggestions for approaching a student athlete suspected of disordered eating:

- The individual (e.g., coach, staff member) who has the best rapport with the student athlete should be the one to approach the athlete, and it should be done in a private setting (e.g., a private meeting).

- In a respectful tone, indicate specific observations that led to the concern, being sure to give the athlete time to respond.

- Choose "I" statements over "you" statements to avoid placing the athlete on the defensive. For example, "I've noticed that you've been fatigued lately, and I'm concerned about you" is preferable to "You need to eat and everything will be fine."

- Avoid giving simple solutions (e.g., "Just eat something") to a complex problem. This will only encourage the student athlete to hide the behavior from you in the future.

- Avoid discussing implications for team participation and instead affirm that the student athlete's role on the team will not be jeopardized by an admission to a problem. The team may be the athlete's only diversion from his or her disordered eating. By eliminating this opportunity for social support and the supervision of a coach or trainer, the athlete may dive into further pathology.

- Regardless of whether the student athlete responds with denial or hostility, it is important to encourage him or her to meet with a professional for an assessment. Acknowledge that seeking outside help is often beneficial and is not a sign of weakness (Hill 2001).

The National Association of Anorexia Nervosa and Associated Disorders (ANAD) created the CONFRONT plan for approaching an individual with an eating disorder that could readily be adapted to the athlete:

- Express **C**oncern for the athlete by saying that you care about his or her mental, physical, and nutritional needs.
- Get **O**rganized; plan where to confront the individual and determine a convenient time.
- Having support groups and eating disorder resources available will be an immediate **N**eed after the confrontation.
- **F**ace the athlete empathetically but directly. Remember to expect denial when you confront him or her.
- Be sure to **R**espond to the athlete by listening to his or her concerns in an athlete-centered manner.
- **O**ffer help and suggestions for how the athlete should proceed, and be willing to support the athlete in the recovery process to ensure that the athlete follows through.
- **N**egotiate another time to talk with the athlete once he or she has sought professional help.
- Finally, recognize that recovery is **T**ime-intensive and that the athlete faces many challenges in the treatment process.

Intervention: Providing Referrals and Arranging for Treatment

Successful intervention requires adequate preparation. To be prepared to help an athlete seek treatment, it is important to develop an eating disorder resource network *before* problems emerge. Individuals and programs specializing in eating disorder treatment should be identified and a list of resources and referrals should be constructed and kept handy. It may even be helpful to distribute the resource list to all athletic support staff. Such a list would have been extremely useful in Cassie's case. The cheerleading coach would likely have felt more comfortable approaching Cassie if she had had a list of referrals or at the very least a contact to recommend.

At the middle and high school levels, a school counselor may be the first contact. If no school counselor is available, check the Yellow Pages or the Web for community resources. At the university level, a college counseling center may offer some specialized resources and support. However, it is important to realize that many generalized mental health facilities are beginning to refer clients with eating disorders to eating disorder specialists or treatment centers across the country. Therefore, do your research in advance so that you are able to provide a direct link to services for your athlete. Some Web sites and books about eating disorders are provided in appendix C.

Managing Diverse Responses to Intervention

Every intervention situation is unique and it is difficult to predict exactly how a given athlete will respond when approached about his or her eating disorder. Coaches and teammates have also been known to demonstrate a variety of responses when learning that a member of the team is suffering from an eating disorder. Thus, successfully managing disordered eating necessitates being familiar with the range of possible responses and the potential impact that they may have on subsequent treatment success (Ryan 1992a).

Athlete's Responses

Upon being confronted about an eating disorder, athletes may exhibit a variety of responses. Some athletes may respond with relief over not having to hide their disorder any longer. This is considered to be the best possible response because it usually means that the athlete will be open and receptive to beginning treatment. Unfortunately, it is also the least common response. The most common responses tend to be denial, anger, and resistance (Ryan 1992a). Just as Michael did, most athletes will deny having an eating disorder or underrate the seriousness of their disordered eating behaviors. They often express anger toward the person who wants to change their behavior out of fear of what those changes may entail (e.g.,

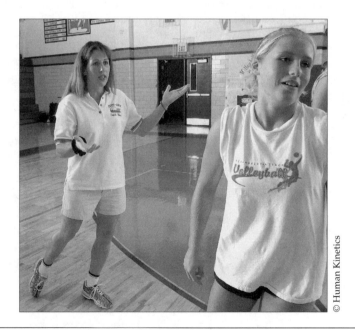

© Human Kinetics

Athletes who fear that their performance will suffer if they discontinue their disordered eating will typically respond defensively when approached and refuse treatment.

weight gain). They steadfastly resist help, believing as many athletes do that they can and should just "tough it out" (Ryan 1992a; Thompson and Sherman 1993; Goldner 1989). Under these circumstances, intervention cannot be successful unless it helps the athlete overcome his or her rationale for opposing medical or therapeutic treatment.

Even if an athlete acknowledges the existence of the eating disorder, he or she may respond defensively when approached and refuse treatment. This response is typically made by athletes who are still performing well and fear that their performance will suffer if they discontinue their disordered eating (Ryan 1992a). Other feelings of hesitancy about receiving treatment may be due to deeper psychological fears, such as fear of losing control over their lives by no longer engaging in rigid eating or exercise behaviors or having to face painful feelings that they had blocked out by focusing on their food intake and weight. The fear may stem from lack of trust of the medical professionals who offer the treatment (Thompson and Sherman 1993). They may doubt the professionals' understanding of their feelings or think that their main objective is to "fatten them up" (Goldner, Birmingham, and Smye 1997).

To reduce the athlete's fears regarding treatment, it is important to provide him or her with a strong sense of autonomy. Letting the athlete know that he or she has a variety of options regarding both the types of treatment received and the health professionals who provide the treatments gives the athlete a feeling of independence and may motivate him or her to explore treatment options (Goldner 1989; Goldner, Birmingham, and Smye 1997).

There are circumstances in which, despite the best possible approach techniques, the athlete refuses treatment. This is a difficult situation, especially if the athlete appears to have developed physical complications from the disorder that affect his or her ability to practice and compete safely. In this case, the coach should call a meeting with the athlete, team physician, and trainer to further express their concerns and convince the athlete to seek treatment (Thompson and Sherman 1993). If the athlete continues to refuse treatment, it is the responsibility of the coach to prohibit the athlete from training and competing with the team (Thompson and Sherman 1993).

Coach's Responses

Like the athlete, coaches are likely to demonstrate a range of responses upon learning that one of their athletes is suffering from an eating disorder. Some coaches will feel disappointment ("I've lost a key player for the season and possibly forever"), others will experience anger ("I've invested a lot of time and energy into this athlete, and now it is wasted!"), and still others will show a complete lack of interest in or disregard for the problem ("What I don't know won't hurt me or the athlete"; "The athlete is performing well so why mess with success?" Ryan 1992a). These responses are difficult to handle and are not particularly conducive to successful treatment of the athlete with disordered eating. Responses such as these dictate that the coach receive counseling along with the athlete.

The best and luckily some of the most common responses from coaches upon learning that one of their athletes is suffering from an eating disorder are concern and compassion. Most coaches want to help the athlete, although all too often they are unsure of what to do. Cassie's cheerleading coach provides a perfect example of a situation in which the coaches' good intentions were stymied by a lack of knowledge in eating disorder intervention. It also demonstrates why it is so important that coaches receive eating disorder education and be prepared to handle the situation should it occur.

More often than not, coaches also experience a degree of guilt when learning that an athlete has an eating disorder (Ryan 1992a). The feeling of culpability generally stems from the belief that he or she could and should have prevented the eating disorder. The coach will likely question his or her role in the disorder's development: "Did I push the athlete too hard?" "Did I put too much pressure on the athlete?" "How could I have missed the warning signs?" Provided that the coach does not feel that others are blaming him or her and become defensive, guilt may be one of the more constructive responses (Ryan 1992a). Generally coaches who harbor a degree of guilt are more open to intervention and more willing to be supportive during the athlete's treatment and recovery.

Teammates' Responses

Teammates' responses reflect the variety of emotions that they experience upon learning that a team member is suffering from an eating disorder. They may experience relief that the athlete will be getting help, which is perhaps the best possible response, as it is likely to generate the most support for the athlete (Ryan 1992a). Other team members may feel guilty, especially if they were aware of their teammate's disorder but did not know how to respond or failed to report it. This response may be particularly conducive to bringing the issue of eating disorders out into the open and providing an opportunity to discuss strategies for eating disorder prevention and intervention (Ryan 1992a). Occasionally, team members will blame the coach or other athletic staff for failing to recognize or react to their teammate's eating disorder. This may inadvertently create a feeling of distrust that may render the athletes reluctant to turn to the coach for help in the future, either for a troubled teammate or themselves.

Another reaction sometimes expressed by team members is fear. They fear that they too might succumb to an eating disorder. Or, if they already suffer from disordered eating behaviors, they may fear being exposed. Teammates may also occasionally feel angry and disappointed in the teammate who has succumbed to an eating disorder and subsequently let the team down (Ryan 1992a). These reactions generally stem from a lack of understanding of the etiology and pathology of eating disorders; thus, education is crucial to allay the fears and contempt of team members and create an environment that is supportive and conducive to the successful treatment of the athlete with disordered eating.

Monitoring Treatment and Follow-Up Care

Although the coach and athletic support staff are not *directly* involved in eating disorder treatment or even posttreatment care, they play important, albeit indirect, roles in both processes. Successful treatment necessitates the support and cooperation of the coach and training staff. The athlete with disordered eating will likely feel embarrassed and ashamed, convinced of the coach's disappointment and disfavor. Understanding and reassurance from the coach is therefore essential to the athlete's recovery. When the coach and athletic staff are committed to being a part of the solution and dedicated to helping the athlete, they can be invaluable to the treatment process (Ryan 1992a).

Successful treatment depends not only on a supportive coaching and training staff but also on the establishment of trust between the athlete and the individuals involved in providing treatment. As previously mentioned, a common reason for an athlete to deny his or her eating disorder or refuse treatment is the shame associated with exposure. Moreover, the athlete is unlikely to open up during treatment, to freely express feelings and emotions if he or she feels that coaches, trainers, or teammates will judge him or her. Thus, confidentiality becomes an important issue during both the treatment and follow-up care of the athlete suffering from disordered eating (Thompson and Sherman 1993).

Maintaining confidentiality can be particularly difficult in the sport setting. The team environment necessitates closeness among the coach, trainers, and team members. Given such an intimate relationship, it is unlikely that the athlete's eating disorder has gone unnoticed, and thus it is equally unlikely that treatment will go unnoticed or proceed without questions. A concerned coach or trainer may want to know how the athlete is progressing in treatment or feel responsible for making sure that he or she is keeping appointments and following treatment protocols. Similarly, members of the team may seek information out of curiosity or concern for their teammate. To protect the athlete with disordered eating as well as avoid legal liability, confidentiality must be established and strictly enforced.

Confidentiality ensures that personal information or details of the athlete's treatment are released to authorized individuals only after the patient has provided written consent (Thompson and Sherman 1993). The ideal situation is for the athlete to sign a release stating that all members of the treatment team and all pertinent members of the coaching and training staff are privy to the treatment protocols and progress of the athlete. Most athletes will agree to this format if they are assured that personal issues relating to the eating disorder will not be discussed (Ryan 1992a).

If the athlete is treated on an outpatient basis, a decision must be made as to whether or not he or she should be allowed to continue to train or compete. Primary to the decision is the athlete's health, both psychological and physical (Ryan 1992a). If training or competition will further jeopardize the athlete's health, a reduction in or, in cases of severe complications, complete discontinuation of training and competition may be warranted. Barring any severe health complications, all those involved with the athlete's treatment must weigh the risks and benefits when negotiating whether an athlete should be allowed to continue to train or compete during treatment.

If an athlete is barred from training or competition during treatment, he or she may become further socially isolated, which could complicate or impede treatment. No longer being a part of the team can contribute to generalized feelings of loss and rejection that may serve to aggravate disordered eating symptoms (Holliman 1991). Allowing the athlete to remain active with the team (albeit with appropriate reductions in training and competition) provides the athlete with an invaluable source of social support and guidance (Thompson and Sherman 1993). Moreover, allowing the athlete to continue to train and compete during treatment may help him or her maintain self-concept and self-esteem as well as provide a sense of hopefulness, all of which may increase his or her motivation to get well. It is generally believed that the more positive the athlete is about treatment, the greater the likelihood that the treatment will be successful (Thompson and Sherman 1993).

Nonetheless, if either the coach or sport participation is contributing to the eating disorder, then discontinuation of training and competition may be necessary. Moreover, if the coach is not supportive of treatment or routinely sends mixed messages to the athlete, then it is probably best that the athlete not train or compete under that particular coach. For example, the athlete may be confused if a coach expresses concern during practice but then pressures the athlete to win at all costs during competition or, as was the case with Cassie, if the athlete receives contradictory messages from different coaches, one expressing concern about the disorder and another almost encouraging it. Finally, continuing to compete may distract the athlete from devoting full attention to treatment. The athlete may use training or competition as an excuse for missing therapy appointments, as a rationalization for deviating from prescribed nutritional plans, or as a justification to train harder or longer than he or she is supposed to (Thompson and Sherman 1993).

Once a decision regarding training and competition during treatment has been agreed upon by the athlete, treatment providers, coach, and athletic trainers, a contract specifying training and competition guidelines should then be created. The contract is designed not only to protect the health of the athlete but also to safeguard those involved in the athlete's treatment. The contract should outline the specific terms and conditions under which the athlete may train and compete (e.g., he or she must maintain a particular body weight, attend all scheduled psychological and nutritional counseling sessions, and be medically evaluated on a regular basis). The athlete should also be closely monitored during treatment by the treatment team for any signs that training or competition is interfering with treatment.

The issue of training and competing must also be addressed during the posttreatment or follow-up period. Like the decision about sport participation during treatment, the decision about the degree of training and competition that the athlete may undertake after treatment should be based on his or her physical, psychological, and emotional health and his or her readiness to return to athletic participation. It is not unusual for an athlete who has completed formal treatment to have some residual psychological issues and to show some lingering disordered eating behaviors or symptoms. If the athlete is still suffering physical complications or severe psychological difficulties or indicates that he or she is not ready to return to training and competition, then he or she should not be allowed to do so. In less clear-cut circumstances, the treatment team along with the coach, athletic trainer, and the athlete must again weigh the risks and benefits and then agree on a plan of action (Thompson and Sherman 1993). A contract similar to that developed during treatment protects the interests of all involved and ensures that the athlete returns to training and competition in the best psychological and physical shape possible.

Cassie and Michael Revisited

This chapter began with two case studies of athletes struggling with disordered eating. Throughout the chapter, references were made to Cassie and Michael to aid in the understanding and application of the material presented. A final word concerning the proper management of these two athletes seems to be an appropriate way to end this chapter. In both cases, management was handled poorly, and the athlete's treatment chances were compromised as a result. A central component of eating disorder management that was not specifically discussed in this chapter but has been emphasized in other chapters is the importance of education. Michael had misperceptions that only females suffer from disordered eating, when in actuality the prevalence has been estimated to be as high as 57% in some male sports. For Michael, education regarding males and eating disorders may have helped render him more receptive to the approach of his teammate. Similarly, Cassie's cheerleading coach probably would have been more apt to approach her if she had known how, if she had received proper education and training regarding how to manage eating disorders in athletes.

Summary

The management of disordered eating in athletes involves identification, approach and referral, treatment support, and post-treatment follow-up. Critical to effective management of disordered eating in athletes is education. Coaches, trainers, and athletic support staff need to know *when* and *how* to approach the athlete with disordered eating and convince him or her to get treatment. They also need to be prepared to arrange treatment by maintaining a list of resources and referrals to eating disorder programs and specialists. Finally, coaches, trainers, and even teammates need to be supportive yet mindful of the athlete's privacy while he or she is in treatment. The guidelines for athletic participation and confidentiality during treatment must be established early on and then strictly enforced.

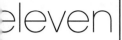

eleven

Successful Eating Disorder Screening, Prevention, and Treatment Programs for Athletes

CHAPTER OBJECTIVES

After reading this chapter, you will be able to

■ describe the essential components of successful eating disorder prevention, screening, and treatment programs, and

■ identify potential roadblocks to eating disorder program development and implementation as well as some strategies for overcoming those roadblocks.

What Characterizes a Successful Eating Disorder Program?

A variety of methods and strategies for identifying, preventing, and treating athletes with disordered eating were presented in the previous four chapters. There is such a variety, in fact, that it may be difficult to determine which strategies should be included in an eating disorder program. Ideally, an eating disorder program should incorporate the most effective screening, prevention, and treatment strategies available. This is no easy task, however, as what qualifies as "most effective" will most likely vary, depending on such factors as the athletic environment, available resources, administrative support, coaches' cooperation, and so on. Moreover, given the budget constraints facing both private and public institutions today, the question typically raised prior to program development and implementation is not what *should* be done but rather what *can* be done given limited resources.

This chapter profiles three successful programs for the identification, prevention, and treatment of eating disorders in athletes:

- The Performance Team at the University of Texas at Austin
- The Student Athlete Wellness Team at the University of Utah
- The Weight Management Program at the University of California–Los Angeles (UCLA)

Unlike previous chapters, this chapter is not based on a scientific review of the literature; rather, it is built around interviews conducted with individuals who have actually developed and implemented eating disorder programs for athletes. These individuals were able to provide invaluable insight and a more personal perspective of the trials and tribulations involved in creating and executing eating disorder programs designed specifically for athletes.

It should be noted that the goal of presenting these profiles is not to provide step-by-step instructions for developing and implementing an eating disorder screening, prevention, and treatment program. Rather, it is meant to provide a framework for program development and implementation by describing the essential components of successful programs, highlighting potential roadblocks to program development and implementation, and providing suggestions for overcoming these roadblocks.

Although all of these programs were implemented on college campuses, it does not mean that they are restricted to this setting. In fact, the eating disorder component of the University of Utah Student Athlete Wellness Team actually grew out of a community program. Conversely, the UCLA Weight Management Program has recently expanded out into the community. Thus, all these programs could be readily adapted to a community environment and could be appropriate for a high school, middle school, or outpatient medical setting.

Eating Disorder Program Profiles

While there are a number of communities, medical centers, and academic institutions that maintain programs for the identification, prevention, or treatment of eating disorders in athletes, very few have attempted to address all three components, and even fewer have accomplished the task successfully. The three eating disorder programs spotlighted in this chapter were chosen because they have effectively integrated all three key program components.

Performance Team, University of Texas at Austin

Originally developed in 1985, the University of Texas at Austin's Performance Team is one of the oldest and most well known *structured* eating disorder identification, prevention, and treatment programs for female athletes. The Performance Team is a model program demonstrating how university administrators, intercollegiate athletic departments, voluntary community professionals, and private industry can successfully work together to construct an eating disorder program within a higher-education setting. The program components and protocols of the Performance Team have been published in numerous texts, spotlighted in several journal articles, and copied by many academic institutions for the simple reason that it has been so successful in its mission of protecting the health and well-being and enhancing the performance of female collegiate athletes (Ryan 1992a; 1992b).

Members of the Performance Team include experts in the fields of orthopedics, endocrinology, exercise physiology, body composition, cardiology, pharmacology, psychology, sociology, allergy and immunology, physical therapy, and athletic training. Through this interdisciplinary approach, the Performance Team assesses the effectiveness of conditioning and training programs in improving performance or reducing the incidence of injury, establishes procedures and protocols for these programs, and researches and develops new applications in the area of female athletes' health and performance.

Since its conception almost 20 years ago, the Performance Team has undergone numerous changes in structure and function. Originally an ad hoc team of health professionals (e.g., select team physicians, mental health experts, and dietitians) who met on a regular basis (at least monthly), the Performance Team no longer exists as an entity separate from the department of athletics. Rather, the Performance Team now includes all those providing care to the athlete and has become part of the regular standard of care provided by the University of Texas at Austin athletic department. According to Randa Ryan, the individual who pioneered the Performance Team, "An athlete with an eating disorder is treated no differently than an athlete with a torn ligament. . . . Disordered eating is now part of the University of Texas standard of care."

Because the Performance Team is no longer a separate program, there is no longer a distinct staff or team of individuals functioning for the specific purpose of addressing eating disorders in athletes. Rather, all those who are involved with athletes are considered part of the team. Nonetheless, the key personnel (i.e., those most often directly involved with the care of athletes with disordered eating) are the team physicians and the university psychologists. Although not always involved in treatment, the university does maintain a dietitian on staff who is available to work with athletes with eating disorders.

Figure 11.1 presents the Performance Team protocol for education about and prevention and treatment of eating disorders in female athletes. It should be noted that this is the original flow chart developed when the Performance Team was first conceived and functioned as a distinct entity. Since the Performance Team encompasses everyone associated with athletes (and not just a distinct group of health and medical professionals) and does not formally review disordered eating cases, the center box (i.e., "Performance Team reviews case and makes recommendations for intervention and treatment") is no longer applicable.

Initial screening for disordered eating is carried out during the preparticipation physical exams. The team physicians, athletic trainers, and gynecologist interview the athletes and examine them for signs and symptoms of disordered eating. According to Dr. Ryan, the physical examination can be a key tool for identifying disordered eating early if the health professional knows what to look for and asks the right questions. Dr Ryan believes that eating disorders are just another indication of psychological distress. Thus, the physician can often look to other psychological issues (e.g., alcohol or drug abuse, depression, other risky behaviors) to help identify disordered eating. Developing a rapport and establishing trust with the athlete is essential for ascertaining honest and accurate information during the preparticipation exam. Dr. Ryan asserts that self-disclosure is a key element to the success of the Performance Team screening program.

Although a validated self-report eating disorder questionnaire was initially part of the interview, the Performance Team no longer utilizes such questionnaires, as research done during the early days of the Team's existence demonstrated that these questionnaires tended to be inaccurate and frequently led to underreporting. Instead, all female athletes complete a comprehensive health history (which includes questions regarding body image, menstrual function, body weight fluctuations, and history of eating disorder diagnosis) and a three-day food log that is reviewed by a dietitian and the team physician for signs of energy and micronutrient inadequacies as well as disordered eating patterns.

Education is the cornerstone of prevention for the Performance Team. Every individual in student services (e.g., coaches, athletic trainers, academic counselors, resident advisors, athletic administrators) receives education regarding disordered eating that includes information about identification (e.g., warning signs and symptoms to watch for), prevention (e.g., how to handle body weight and dieting issues), and treatment (e.g., how to approach and refer an athlete suspected of disordered eating). All newly hired athletic personnel are required to attend a series of eating

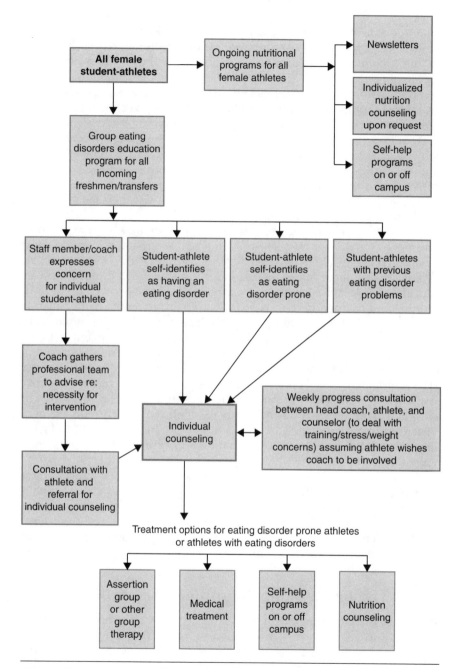

Figure 11.1 Performance Team protocol for education about and prevention and treatment of eating disorders. Counseling includes psychological and nutritional counseling.

Reprinted, by permission, from R. Ryan, 1992, Management of eating problems in the athletic setting. In *Eating, bodyweight and performance in athletes: Disorders of modern society,* edited by K. Brownell, J. Rodin, and J.H. Wilmore (Philadelphia, PA: Lippincott, Williams, and Wilkins), 354.

disorder educational sessions early in their employment. In addition, all athletic personnel receive updated educational materials regularly and are required to attend periodic refresher courses on eating disorder prevention and treatment.

The university also maintains very strict policies regarding body weight and weight control practices. For example, no coach is allowed to interact with a student athlete regarding body weight. Similarly, no coach is allowed to prescribe diets to or give advice on weight loss strategies. Coaches and athletic personnel are, however, expected to be sensitive to weight issues and encouraged to maintain an open atmosphere regarding disordered eating. According to Dr. Ryan, the key to successful prevention efforts lies in "creating a family environment with coaches and teams, one in which it is OK to talk about disordered eating."

There is no standardized treatment protocol; rather, treatment is handled on an individual, case-by-case basis. That is, if an athlete is identified with disordered eating, she is evaluated by the team physician and a staff psychologist, who then determine her course of treatment. The team physician also decides whether or not the athlete should be allowed to continue training and competing, a decision that is largely governed by the severity of the disorder and the degree to which the athlete's health is or could be compromised. For example, a bulimic athlete who engages in binge–purge cycles on a daily basis and demonstrates electrolyte imbalances would be barred from both training and competition. On the other hand, a bulimic athlete who binges and purges once a week and shows no signs of electrolyte imbalances (or other manifestations of compromised health) would be allowed to continue to train and compete, albeit at a slightly reduced level. That is, training time and intensity would be reduced, as would playing time in competition (team sports) or number of competitive events (individual sports).

According to Dr. Ryan, most cases of disordered eating in athletes have been treated on an outpatient basis, and very few athletes were completely withheld from training or competition. This is largely due to the proactive nature of their screening and identification program. That is, disordered eating is identified and treated early on in the progression of the disorder, and thus the physiological and psychological consequences tend to be less severe.

Student Athlete Wellness Team, University of Utah

The eating disorder program at the University of Utah has been in existence for nearly six years. The program actually grew out of a community-based eating disorder treatment program that was developed by Dr. Elizabeth Joy. As the team physician for the University of Utah, Dr. Joy noted that the athletics department was experiencing difficulty tracking athletes with disordered eating. The university did not maintain a formal screening for disordered eating among the athletic population. As a result, a significant number of athletes who were suffering from disordered eating were not receiving timely or appropriate care. Thus, Dr. Joy offered to adapt her community-based eating disorder program to the university setting. Soon thereafter, the program became a pivotal part of the university's Student Athlete Wellness Team, a multidisciplinary team consisting of the team physician, a sport nutritionist, a mental health professional, and select athletic trainers.

The eating disorder program component of the Student Athlete Wellness Team is comprehensive and includes screening (identification), prevention, and treatment components (Joy et al. 1997a; 1997b). Screening for disordered eating is accomplished by having every incoming female freshman athlete complete a self-report questionnaire on eating and body weight (see appendix F for the full questionnaire) and be interviewed in depth by a sport nutritionist during the preparticipation physicals. The questionnaire and interview ascertain information regarding the athlete's menstrual function, weight history, dieting or methods of weight control, and typical food intake. In addition to the interview conducted by the sport nutritionist, the team physician questions all female athletes about diet and nutrition during their preparticipation physical exam.

Prevention efforts center on nutrition education, which is provided largely by the sport nutritionist on staff. Topics discussed either in group sessions (i.e., team presentations) or individual counseling sessions include the general components of a healthful diet, sport-specific nutritional guidelines for training and competition, and any other information requested by either the athletes or coaches. The individual counseling sessions with athletes are thought to be particularly useful in identification and early intervention of disordered eating. Dr. Joy asserts that individual consultations with the sport nutritionist often serve as a "second line of defense" in confirming suspected cases of disordered eating or those that may have been missed during the preparticipation physical.

The Student Athlete Wellness Team takes a multidisciplinary approach to the treatment of disordered eating in athletes. In the outpatient setting the team consists of a sport nutritionist, a variety of mental health professionals who are either clinical psychologists or licensed clinical social workers, and a physician who is board certified in family practice and has a certificate of added qualification in sports medicine. Additionally, the Student Athlete Wellness Team includes a representative (a certified athletic trainer; ATC) from the athletic training department, the head or associate strength coach, and one of the associate athletic directors (Joy et al. 1997a). According to Dr. Joy, treatment is generally done on an outpatient basis, except in severe or difficult-to-treat cases. During treatment, athletes may be restricted from training or competition if the Student Athlete Wellness Team believes that their health will be negatively affected by participation. For example, if an athlete drops below a minimally acceptable body weight or experiences chest pain, palpitations, syncope, or repeated near syncope, she will most likely be restricted from both training and competition. Similarly, an athlete is restricted from athletic participation if a physical examination reveals electrocardiogram abnormalities, electrolyte abnormalities, or any other abnormalities consistent with starvation or bingeing and purging.

Weight Management Program, University of California-Los Angeles

The eating disorder program at the University of California–Los Angeles (UCLA) is a component of the UCLA Weight Management Program and has been in existence for over 10 years. A medical team that includes team physicians, athletic trainers, sport psychologists, a sport nutritionist, and a psychiatrist (when necessary or appropriate) administers the UCLA Weight Management Program. Dr. Aurelia Nattiv, a UCLA team physician and the individual who was largely responsible for the program's development and implementation, reported that the UCLA Weight Management Program did not materialize overnight. Rather, it developed gradually over time as more and more female athletes presented with disordered eating problems. Moreover, the program has not remained static but has been modified and enhanced each year as a result of feedback from medical and athletic personnel as well as the athletes themselves (Nattiv and Lynch 1994; Nattiv et al. 1994).

Like the other two eating disorder programs described, the UCLA Weight Management Program maintains protocols (with some flexibility) for screening, prevention, and treatment of eating disorders in athletes. Team physicians screen all female athletes for disordered eating and menstrual dysfunction at the time of their annual preparticipation physical. The screening instrument used is a modified version of the preparticipation questionnaire used by the American Academy of Family Physicians (AAFP) and the American Medical Society for Sports Medicine (AMSSM; see appendix F). The modifications include a more in-depth menstrual history and additional questions on body image, dieting practices, and weight loss history. If any of the responses indicate disordered eating, further inquiry is made by the physician. According to Dr. Nattiv, all team physicians are trained to recognize the warning signs and symptoms of disordered eating. Athletes identified during the preparticipation exam as being at risk for disordered eating receive a follow-up exam by the head team physician (Dr. Nattiv) or the physician assigned to the athlete's team. The follow-up exam consists of additional physical, biochemical, nutritional tests, and sometimes psychological assessments. If the athlete is diagnosed with an eating disorder on the basis of the additional workup, she is assigned to ongoing management, which involves periodic physical exams and nutritional as well as psychological counseling, the frequency of which depend on the severity of the disorder.

Prevention efforts are also carried out by the team physicians and involve educational programming for coaches, trainers, and other athletic personnel. The education consists of seminars, videos, and reading materials on disordered eating in athletes. In addition, both team educational sessions on nutrition and individual nutritional counseling are available for the athletes.

One of the key elements of the UCLA Weight Management Program is the strict policy concerning body weight assessment. In fact, the Weight Management Program maintains a specific protocol regarding the assessment of body weight, including who is qualified to assess body weight, what type of assessments are permitted, and how the assessments may be utilized. According to the protocol, all issues regarding body weight or body composition are to be addressed *only* by the medical team in strict confidentiality with the athlete. Coaches are forbidden from commenting on weight issues to or about athletes, conducting team or group weigh-ins, singling out an individual athlete for weighing, or recommending weight loss to an athlete.

The protocol is enforced with the help of athlete mentors and athletic trainers, who monitor coaches for any potential violations, such as a coach's requesting a weigh-in, pressuring an athlete to lose weight, or providing improper weight loss advice. If a violation occurs, the coach is issued a warning (which goes on his or her record) and is required to meet with the team physician or athletic trainer to review the components and purpose of the protocol and the boundaries set forth by it. Any concerns that the coach may have regarding an athlete's weight are then referred to the medical team for management or further exploration.

Similar to the University of Utah program, treatment is done on an individual, case-by-case basis and generally follows a team approach, involving the appropriate members of the medical team (any or all of the following: team physician, psychologist or psychiatrist, and sport dietitian). The medical team meets monthly to review new cases and evaluate the progress of existing cases.

A contract outlining treatment expectations is often used with high-risk athletes (i.e., those with more severe eating disorders and/or a history of management difficulty) so that both the medical team and the athlete have a clear understanding of the steps needed for the athlete to compete safely or for the athlete's health to improve so that competition can be resumed). The contract clearly delineates the frequency of required appointments with the team physician, sport dietitian, and psychologist or psychiatrist. It states whether the athlete has a weight cutoff that she must stay above in order to train or compete. If the athlete does not comply with one or more of the contract's requirements or shows no sign of improvement or evidence of deterioration, then her ability to train or compete is reevaluated. See appendix G for an example of this type of contract.

Roadblocks to Program Implementation

All three of the individuals interviewed for this chapter indicated that developing their eating disorder programs (i.e., devising program components) was far less complicated than actually implementing them. According to Drs. Joy, Nattiv, and Ryan, the path to program implementation was lined with a variety of roadblocks. The most formidable roadblock, according to the program developers, was lack of support or outright resistance from the athletic administration. For those familiar with both disordered eating and the nature of athletic governance, this should come as no surprise. Disordered eating is a delicate, frequently controversial, and often poorly understood topic, with potentially serious legal ramifications. Thus, it is understandable that the athletic administration would be wary of or even outright resistant to the implementation of programs designed to address disordered eating, particularly if the programs are developed or implemented by individuals outside the athletic administration hierarchy.

At the heart of the typical administration's reluctance to embrace an eating disorder program is unease with relinquishing control. According to UCLA's Dr. Nattiv, "Giving up control [over a portion of the athlete's care] was what the administration feared most." At the University of Utah, one of the greatest challenges faced by the Student Athlete Wellness Team also was convincing the athletic administration to relinquish the responsibility of managing disordered eating. Dr. Joy reported: "We had to *prove* to the athletic administration that we were knowledgeable, competent, and had the best interest of the athletes at heart."

A perhaps less formal but equally formidable roadblock were the coaches. Once again the difficulty seemed to come down to the issue of control and the ramifications of losing that control. The coach is ultimately responsible for the performance of his or her athletes; thus, they are likely to be resistant to the idea of turning over weight management and disordered eating issues to the medical team. In Dr. Nattiv's experience, many coaches either initially refused the services (particularly the nutrition and eating disorder education) offered by the medical team, or they would reluctantly comply but either would not reinforce the information or would act in direct opposition to the suggestions provided. However, Dr. Nattiv noted that eventually she and her team were able to wear down the coaches' resistance. In her own words, "Once the coaches were able to see the outcomes of the program, they were better able to appreciate its benefits, and the resistance gradually subsided."

Dr. Ryan's experience with the coaches was somewhat different. Most were open to the Performance Team's interventions; in fact, some coaches actually "breathed a sigh of relief" when the responsibility of managing disordered eating was removed from their shoulders and placed on those of the Performance Team. It's no wonder. Coaches have historically shouldered the bulk of the blame for the development of disordered eating in their athletes. Thus, removing the responsibility of weight control issues from the coaches also eases the burden of blame for weight-related disorders that may develop among their athletes.

Athletes can also create barriers to the implementation of an eating disorder program. As Dr. Ryan explained, "Athletes can be a highly resistant group. . . . Yet without the support of the student athletes, the program cannot get off the ground, and even if it did it would likely have little impact." Just like the coaches (or perhaps because of them), many athletes were initially hesitant and sometimes openly opposed to the programs offered to them by the Performance Team, particularly those that dealt directly with eating disorders. The topic tended to make athletes feel uneasy, particularly those suffering from disordered eating, as they feared discovery and the resulting ramifications. Unfortunately, without the athlete's support the program will be largely ineffective. Athletes have to be open to and willing to adopt the proposed programs and the medical and nutritional recommendations provided by them.

Other challenges reported by Drs. Joy, Nattiv, and Ryan included organizing and assembling members of the team and figuring out alternative ways to compensate team members for their time and effort. While some team members are employees of the university or contract workers paid on a fee-for-service basis, many are not paid any additional stipend for their work on the eating disorder team but rather volunteer their time as a community service. Thus, it can be difficult to gather professionals of the quality necessary for an effective team. A final challenge reported was that of regularly refining and updating the program so as to keep it current and able to meet the needs of a diverse and ever-changing student-athlete population.

Keys to Successful Eating Disorder Programs

As demonstrated in the previous section, the roadblocks to program development and implementation faced by Drs. Joy, Nattiv, and Ryan were strikingly similar. It thus should not be surprising that their advice for breaking down those barriers was also quite similar. According to the program developers, the keys to successfully implementing an eating disorder program are allaying the fears and securing the trust of the athletic administrators, coaches, and athletes.

Gaining Support of the Athletic Administration

The first step in gaining the support of the athletic administration is to allay their fears of loss of control. As Dr. Ryan explained, "The administrative staff needs to be assured that they are not *losing* control of the athletes but rather *gaining* the support of a team of experts that are duly qualified to manage athletes at risk for or suffering from disordered eating." This can best be accomplished by both providing the administration with evidence of the eating disorder team's expertise and involving the administration in the development and implementation of the eating disorder program. Evidence of the team's expertise can be demonstrated by providing statements of credentials, securing letters of recommendation, and supplying a curriculum vitae or other description of the team members' experience in the area of disordered eating. The administration can be involved in many areas of program development and implementation, including designing program components, creating program protocols, and identifying and assembling team members.

Once the eating disorder program is implemented, it is crucial to maintain open lines of communication between the eating disorder team and the athletic administration. Having at least one athletic administrator serve as a member of the eating disorder team not only allows the administration to have input but also provides a mechanism for communication between the team and the administration.

Achieving Acceptance by Coaches

Once approval has been granted by the athletic administration, the next step in successful program implementation is to get the coaches on board. As previously mentioned, coaches may be somewhat more resistant to eating disorder programs than the administration because they are directly responsible for their athletes and, thus, they have a greater stake in the outcomes. The tactics for achieving the coaches' acceptance of the eating disorder program are similar to those previously described for the athletic administration and include (1) convincing coaches of the eating disorder team's expertise, (2) involving them in program development and implementation, and (3) maintaining open lines of communication. However, the *specific* strategies for carrying out these tactics are somewhat more complex. For example, statements of the medical and nutritional professionals' credentials are generally of lesser importance in convincing coaches of their expertise than knowledge of the professionals' reputations, positive recommendations (particularly from other coaches), and personal experience with them. Indeed, for coaches, seeing (or hearing) is believing. Thus, it is imperative that all members of the team strive to make a good first impression with the coach and make every effort to openly demonstrate their expertise.

The level of involvement in program development and implementation will also be greater for the coaches compared to the athletic administration. Coaches are generally more willing to embrace an eating disorder program if they feel a sense of ownership for that program. Thus, coaches should be intricately involved in both program development and implementation. In fact, the very nature of the coaches' relationship with and proximity to their athletes renders them invaluable to implementing a successful eating disorder program. They are on the front lines, so to speak. They know best what kinds of issues plague their athletes, how to most effectively communicate with their athletes, and how to successfully motivate their athletes. Thus, they can identify which program components are most important and most likely to be effective for preventing and identifying eating disorders in their athletes.

Education is also essential in gaining the coaches' trust and endorsement for an eating disorder program. Often coaches' resistance stems from a lack of knowledge or understanding of disordered eating. Thus, providing educational opportunities for coaches (e.g., holding seminars that cover such topics as disordered eating, sport nutrition, and healthful weight management) is an important first step toward breaking down the barriers of resistance.

Finally, maintaining open lines of communication between the coaches and members of the eating disorder team is crucial. Coaches are in a prime position to monitor their athletes' behaviors and reactions. They know, for example, if the educational components of the eating disorder prevention program are taking hold and sinking in. They know whether the prevention components of the program are working. Thus, coaches should be contacted and consulted regularly (i.e., at least monthly, if not weekly) by team members to ensure that they understand and approve of the programs, policies, and procedures and are content with its outcomes. Coaches should have ample opportunity to pose questions and express concerns to team members. Similarly, team members should feel comfortable communicating any concerns or questions regarding the coaches' training policies or other actions that affect the athletes.

It should be noted that coaches may have difficulty discussing sensitive issues related to disordered eating either with eating disorder team members or with athletes. This sensitivity generally arises from coaches' feelings of culpability for athletes' disordered eating behaviors. While there are probably still some instances in which a coach directly contributes to an athlete's disordered eating, most coaches today are well aware of the liabilities involved and are very careful not to overstep their boundaries regarding weight and dieting issues. Thus, it is important to avoid placing blame. Coaches need to be held accountable for their athletes in a way that is not threatening. According to Dr. Ryan, the best way to do this is to make disordered eating a "health and safety issue, not a coaching issue."

Winning Over the Athletes

As previously described, an eating disorder screening, prevention, and treatment program cannot be effective if the athletes do not buy in to it. Thus, enlisting the athletes' support is essential for successful program implementation. Once again, the coaches play a pivotal role. Coaches can either rally the athletes behind the program or turn them against it. In other words, if the coach endorses the program, chances are his or her athletes will follow suit. Dr. Ryan suggests creating a shared perception of disordered eating, its causes and consequences, and its prevention and treatment among the athletes, coaches, and eating disorder team members. Team educational sessions and open forums for discussion of sensitive issues (e.g., eating, body weight, and performance) are the best way to create this shared perception. All three eating disorder programs profiled in this chapter utilize and have experienced great success with team educational sessions and focused discussion groups.

Creating a Cohesive Eating Disorder Team

No eating disorder program can be successful without a committed and cohesive team. Members of the eating disorder team must be supportive of one another and of the program itself. The best way to foster a cohesive team environment is to encourage open communication among team members. According to Dr. Joy, "Open lines of communication between all members of the team is essential, and creating a forum to allow this communication to take place is the best way to keep those lines open." The model of communication used by Dr. Joy and the University of Utah Student Athlete Wellness Team is shown in figure 11.2. More specifically, the diagram depicts the relationship that should ideally exist between the team and the patient (i.e., the student athlete with disordered eating). In this particular model the patient is in the center (i.e., "patient centered") and thus is the focus of treatment by the surrounding health care professionals (i.e., the team physician, nutritionist or dietitian, and mental health provider). For treatment to be effective, the lines of communication (represented in the diagram by arrows) must flow not only between patient and health care providers but also among the health care providers. According to Dr. Joy, "Regular communication between health care providers allows the team to present a united approach, avoids sending contradictory messages, and provides the best opportunity to help the patient in his or her recovery."

Communication between members of the eating disorder team can take many forms but generally consists of team members' open access to writ-

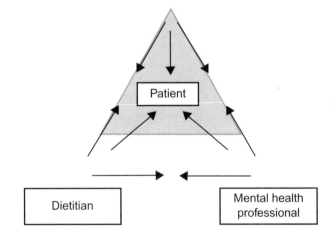

Figure 11.2 Model of communication among members of the eating disorder team and the patient. The arrows represent the various lines of communication. Ongoing communication among all providers allows a united approach to treatment and avoids sending contradictory messages.

Reprinted, by permission, from Elizabeth Joy, University of Utah.

ten reports from each health care provider detailing the patient's progress and periodic team meetings during which patient cases can be discussed and evaluated by all members of the team. In the programs profiled here, members of the team meet at least once a month, and sometimes as often as once a week, to evaluate new eating disorder cases and review the progress and management of existing cases.

Of course, the eating disorder team should be composed of individuals who are experts in and experienced with disordered eating, particularly in athletes. In addition, team members must have the dedication necessary to maintain the eating disorder program. Balancing the expertise of each individual team member while maintaining the cohesiveness of the team can be a challenge in itself. As long as there is sufficient team leadership, however, this challenge is one that can be easily met. As Dr. Joy explained, "Each individual on the team should have [his or her] own domain (that is, area of specialization); however, there is often a fair amount of overlap. . . . It is the responsibility of the team leader to manage this overlap in such a way that no one's ego gets bruised and that each and every person on the team recognizes that they are working toward the common goal of making the athlete better."

Summary

Three successful eating disorder programs—the Performance Team (University of Texas at Austin), the Student Athlete Wellness Team (University of Utah), and the Weight Management Program (UCLA)—were presented in this chapter. The individuals responsible for the conception and implementation of these programs—Dr. Randa Ryan, Dr. Elizabeth Joy, and Dr. Aurelia Nattiv—were interviewed to provide insight into what it takes to successfully develop and implement an eating disorder screening, prevention, and treatment program.

As demonstrated in the chapter, the road to successful program development and implementation was lined with various roadblocks posed by the athletic administration, the coaches, and even the athletes themselves. Nonetheless, through creativity and perseverance, all managed to overcome these obstacles.

According to the individuals interviewed in the chapter, the key to successful development and implementation of eating disorder programs is gaining the trust and support of the athletic administration, coaches, and athletes. The essential elements for gaining that support are communication, education, and a shared perception. Finally, patience and persistence are crucial. Developing and implementing a successful eating disorder program takes work; it requires commitment, persistence, and lots of patience. Nonetheless, the rewards—healthy, happy, and highly successful athletes—are invaluable.

Disordered Eating Case Studies

Case Study 1: Anorexia Nervosa

Jill was a collegiate distance runner. As a freshman she was a mediocre runner, routinely placing fifth or sixth for the team in meets. At the end of her freshman season, her coach mentioned that she might improve her times (and standing on the team) if she were to lose some weight; she did not, however, provide Jill with information or guidance on weight loss.

Jill wanted to be the best runner she could be, so she began her summer vacation determined to lose weight. Jill started by cutting out sweets and other junk foods from her diet. She dropped about 5 lb (2.3 kg) in about four weeks, and friends and family commented on how good she looked. Jill felt lighter when she ran, and her times in a couple of local road races were pretty good, although not good enough. She thought that if she lost just a little more weight, she would perform even better. Jill decided to become a little more restrictive in her eating habits. She stopped eating meat (because she had heard it was fattening) and diligently worked to cut out all sources of fat from her diet. She also severely restricted the amount of breads, grains, and cereals she consumed because she had heard that carbohydrates also make people fat.

As a result of the additional restrictions, Jill's weight dropped fairly quickly; she lost an additional 20 lb (9.1 kg) in just under two months. When Jill returned for the fall cross-country season, she weighed in at 105 lb (47.6 kg) at 5 ft 6 1/2 in. (169 cm) and quickly assumed the position of lead runner on the team. She was setting personal bests in her races and training harder and better than ever before. Despite her improved performance (or perhaps because of it), Jill continued to diet. In fact, her list of allowed foods continued to shrink, until her diet consisted primarily of fruits, vegetables, and an occasional grain product. She also began to exercise on the side, going to the gym after practice and on the weekends to use the stair climber and stationary bike. Jill isolated herself from her teammates and routinely avoided social functions with the team, particularly if they involved eating. Jill's coach and teammates expressed concern for her increasingly emaciated appearance, yet despite their comments and concerns, Jill still felt fat, particularly in her hips and thighs. Even the cessation of her menstrual periods and regular abdominal pain and bloating (particularly late at night) did not dissuade Jill from her continued quest for thinness.

Just three weeks into the season, Jill began to have trouble finishing her workouts, particularly her speed training. She was constantly fatigued, her legs constantly sore. She also started to feel pain just behind her second toe on her right foot. The pain became excruciating, and she was forced to seek medical attention. The diagnosis was a stress fracture in her second metatarsal; the treatment plan was eight weeks of rest.

Needless to say, rest was the last thing Jill felt she could afford. How could she keep her weight down without running? Jill quickly took up other forms of exercise in place of running. She swam, ran in the water, and cycled several hours each day. At the same time, Jill restricted her food intake even more, limiting herself to just 500 kcal/d. Because Jill was not practicing with the team and refused to go to the cafeteria with her teammates for meals, she became more and more isolated from her friends. She did not go home on weekends anymore because she was tired of listening to her parents' chastising comments and seeing their worried faces. Jill's life basically consisted of going to class, studying, exercising, and thinking constantly about the food she would not, could not, eat. Her entire being was focused on controlling her weight, which had now plummeted to 85 lb (38.6 kg).

Jill tried to get back to running several times but was continually plagued by injuries. By her junior year she had lost her cross-country and track scholarship and was not invited back to the team. These setbacks only served to fuel Jill's drive for thinness. Throughout her junior year she continued to restrict her food intake to under 500 kcal/d and to exercise excessively (sometimes five hours a day). She began to develop additional medical symptoms. She frequently complained of being weak and lethargic and was often cold. She developed dry skin and brittle nails, and her hair began to fall out. Jill also noticed that her heartbeat had become very slow (which she attributed to her cardiovascular fitness) and would skip beats occasionally.

One afternoon while working out in the gym (in the middle of a three-hour ride on the stationary bike), Jill began to feel light-headed and experienced a sharp pain in her chest, then everything went black. When she awoke, she was lying in a hospital bed looking up at the concerned faces of her parents. She had suffered an acute myocardial infarction, a heart attack, at the tender age of 22. The realization that she had a problem hit her as hard and as swiftly as the heart attack. When the attending physician recommended that Jill see a psychologist on the staff, she agreed without hesitation. She was exhausted both physically and mentally. She was tired of exercising, tired of counting rice cakes, tired of worrying about her weight; she just wanted to live a normal life.

Jill was diagnosed with anorexia nervosa. She received inpatient treatment for her disorder while recovering in the hospital and began outpatient counseling as soon as she was released. After a year of intensive therapy,

Jill feels she is on the road to recovery. She knows that she will continue to struggle with her disorder for many years, perhaps for the rest of her life, but she admits that she can finally see the light at the end of the tunnel. She is determined to overcome her disorder.

Comment

Jill's plight is common among female athletes who develop anorexia nervosa. The etiology, progression, and consequences of her disorder are characteristically seen in both athletes and nonathletes. Jill's disorder began with a period of dieting (sparked by a desire to improve performance) that became increasingly restrictive and pathogenic. The disorder really took hold when Jill suffered an injury and was no longer able to train (and burn calories) as she had when she was running. As was shown in chapter 3, the impetus for Jill's dieting and the progression of her food restriction are quite common among athletes who develop disordered eating.

The progression of Jill's eating disorder is also a classic example of the development of anorexia nervosa in athletes, particularly female athletes. As Jill's disorder progressed, her list of acceptable foods dwindled, and her obsession with weight grew to epic proportions. In fact, far from being satisfied with her weight loss, it seemed to drive her dieting behaviors. That is, the more weight Jill lost, the more restrictive her eating became. Jill also began to incorporate additional exercise into her grueling dieting regimen.

The consequences, both physical and psychological, suffered by Jill are also characteristic of those seen in athletes with anorexia nervosa (reported in chapters 5 and 6). One of the first symptoms Jill developed was menstrual dysfunction. She later began experiencing chronic abdominal bloating, gastrointestinal pain, and chronic fatigue. Jill developed dry skin, brittle nails, lanugo, alopecia (hair loss), bradycardia, and irregular heartbeats, all common symptoms of the starvation associated with anorexia nervosa. Her performance in both training and competition began to deteriorate, and she was plagued by injuries.

The denial and rationalizations that Jill demonstrated are classic reactions of individuals with eating disorders. As described in chapter 1, despite marked weight loss, significant emotional distress, and severe health problems, individuals with anorexia nervosa deny their disorder to the bitter end or, as in Jill's case, until a significant medical incident occurs. It takes a near-death experience for many people with eating disorders to admit to their disorder and seek or accept treatment. If Jill is a typical anorexic, she will likely require several months or even years of treatment and, like alcoholics, will never be fully cured but rather will always be recovering.

Case Study 2: Bulimia Nervosa

Amy was a 24-year-old competitive triathlete who dreamed of making the U.S. Olympic triathlon team. She also dreamed of the day when she would be able to conquer her addiction to bingeing and purging. Amy had been battling bulimia for five years.

Amy had never been a particularly small girl, nor was she ever *severely* overweight, but she was never as thin or as lean as her competitors. Thus, she had always been unhappy with her body weight. Like many triathletes, Amy came from a swimming background. She started swimming competitively when she was just seven years old, swam in the Amateur Athletic Union (AAU) throughout junior and senior high school, and received a scholarship to swim at the state university. Amy recalled the humiliation of weekly weigh-ins by her coach during both her junior and senior high school swim seasons. If she was over her assigned weight, she was labeled a member of the "fat club," which meant she was forced to sit on the side of the pool, wearing a T-shirt labeled "fat club member," while her teammates practiced. Needless to say, these punitive measures only served to fuel Amy's obsession with weight and exacerbate her negative body image and low self-esteem. During these low points, Amy would often comfort herself with her favorite foods (ice cream, cookies, cake, and candy); however, she would frequently eat too much and was left feeling angry and disgusted with herself. Despite her overeating episodes, Amy did not gain a significant amount of weight (<10 lb, or 4.5 kg), largely because she would always exercise extra hard and restrict her food intake for several days after her binges.

During high school, Amy experimented with a number of different weight loss techniques. She tried juice fasts, total fasts, liquid diets, the cabbage soup diet, and low-carbohydrate diets. She even tried diet pills once, but they just made her jittery and unable to fall asleep at night. Each diet afforded Amy some degree of weight loss (5-10 lb, or 2.3-4.5 kg), but she could never stick to them and thus would typically gain the weight back (often with a few extra pounds). During the summer before her first year of college, Amy decided to get serious about her weight loss; she joined a commercial weight loss program with her mother. Amy was able to drop 15 lb (6.8 kg) in three months; however she still felt fat, despite her parents' and friends' assertions to the contrary.

Amy swam on a partial scholarship her freshman year (she was told she could earn a full scholarship for the following year if she could significantly improve her performance over the course of the season). She had a decent season, but not good enough to earn a full scholarship. She blamed her poor performance on her weight gain. The "freshman 10" actually ended up being the "freshman 20" for Amy. Feeling completely disgusted with herself, she went back to the commercial weight loss program during the summer between her freshman and sophomore years and lost 35 lb (15.9 kg). When she returned to school for her sophomore year, she was determined to keep the weight off and have the best swim season ever.

Amy embarked on a very restrictive diet. She would eat nothing before morning practice, have a granola bar or bagel and a piece of fruit between her morning and afternoon practice, and for dinner would eat only a salad or a small amount of pasta with cooked vegetables. Not surprisingly, her restrictive eating habits left her hungry, moody, and tired. Late one night, after only two weeks on her diet and ravenous from a particularly strenuous afternoon workout, Amy ate a homemade brownie from a batch that her roommate's mother had baked. It tasted so good that she had another, and another, and another. Before she knew it, she had consumed the whole batch (about 24 brownies). Amy was overcome with a sense of panic. She was disgusted with herself for doing such a thing and nauseated from eating so much food so quickly. All she could think about was getting rid of the food she had eaten so that she would not gain back the weight she had worked so hard to lose. She had read an article in a magazine about women who made themselves throw up; at the time she had thought she could never actually do it. Being alone, angry, and anxious, however, she tried it. Amy was amazed at how easy it was. Moreover, once she had vomited, she felt an incredible sense of relief; it was both physically and psychologically cathartic.

This one episode started a seemingly endless cycle of restricting, bingeing, and purging. Initially, Amy binged and purged only a couple of times a week, when she could no longer maintain a restrictive eating pattern. However, soon she was bingeing and purging every day, sometimes as often as three or four times a day, especially during stressful periods such as midterms or swimming finals. Furthermore, she began to purge even when she had eaten just a small amount of food. In fact, as the bulimia progressed, the size of the meal no longer seemed to matter. Any time Amy ate, she felt the need to get rid of the food. The vomiting was taking a toll on her digestive system, causing constant abdominal pain and frequent constipation. The constipation made her feel bloated, so Amy began taking laxatives to regulate her bowel movements. Soon Amy was taking laxatives every day, doubling the dosage just to stay regular. She needed them, just as she needed her bingeing and purging rituals.

The bulimia began to take over Amy's life. Her bulimic practices became more important than school, swimming, or her friends and family. The bulimia began to take an increasing physical toll on Amy as well. She found it hard to get up for morning practice because she felt so washed out. She tried pushing through her workouts but frequently had to quit early because of fatigue or horrible muscle cramps in her legs. She always had a sore throat and red, swollen eyes. Amy eventually had to quit the swim team; the workouts became too taxing, and it was becoming more difficult to hide her bulimic behaviors from her teammates.

Few suspected that Amy had a problem; she was adept at hiding her bingeing and purging behaviors, and she always had a ready excuse for her swollen eyes and face (e.g., she had stayed up late studying, she had trouble with her contact lenses). Nonetheless, her physical symptoms were becoming so severe that even she could no longer ignore them. She had episodes of dizziness, constant stomach pain, and frequent rapid and irregular heartbeats. She had also begun to vomit blood regularly. She knew that she needed medical attention but was reluctant to go to the health center for fear that her secret would be revealed. Amy felt trapped.

It took a particularly bad purging episode, in which Amy could not stop the bleeding from her nose and mouth, to finally convince her to seek medical treatment. She was diagnosed with an esophageal ulcer. In addition, her blood tests indicated that she was anemic and her electrolytes were completely out of balance. The attending physician had had some experience with bulimic patients before and recognized Amy's symptoms. He was able to convince Amy to see a counselor with the university psychological service.

Amy attended counseling sessions for the remainder of her junior year. Unfortunately, the counseling focused more on the pathology of the eating disorder than on the overall place of the disorder in Amy's life and the thought processes that had led her there. (Of course, the counseling may have been more successful had Amy allowed it to be!) The counseling was effective in curtailing her bingeing and purging behaviors. Nonetheless, as Amy later learned, even though the physical manifestations of the eating disorder (i.e., vomiting, using laxatives, excessive exercise) may taper, if the disordered thinking remains, the disorder also remains.

During her senior year of college, Amy took up running because she found that running helped her keep her weight down more than swimming, although she still continued to swim regularly. Amy saw a flyer for a local triathlon and thought it sounded fun. Amy entered the race and placed second in her age category. She really enjoyed it, and so she began to train specifically for the triathlon. Soon Amy was competing regularly. She seemed to excel at the sport and was equally competent in the shorter (sprint) distances and the longer (Olympic) distances. Amy was a natural on the bike (she was sure it was because of her "huge" thighs), and of course, she was a strong swimmer. Her weakest event was the run.

She noticed that the really good female triathletes were a lot thinner than she was, particularly in the hips and thighs. She decided that if she were going to be really competitive in the triathlon and have a shot at the Olympic team, she would have to trim down her legs so that she could run faster. Thus, Amy began to diet. After a month of severe energy restriction and excessive exercise, Amy found herself once again caught in the downward spiral of bingeing and purging. Luckily, this time Amy had a friend who not only recognized her disorder but also ultimately would be instrumental in Amy's intervention and treatment.

Amy met Jennifer through a local triathlon club. They began to train together and soon became good friends. Jennifer noticed that Amy's body weight as well as her moods would fluctuate rapidly and rather dramatically. She also took note of Amy's frequent self-deprecating remarks about her body weight and her excessive training, which seemed to correspond to the amount she had eaten that day. Jennifer had a sister who had suffered from bulimia nervosa and suspected that Amy might be struggling with the same disorder. Jennifer's suspicions were confirmed when she and

Amy went for a pizza after a particularly strenuous evening training run. Amy finished off half a large pizza rather quickly and then immediately excused herself to the bathroom.

Having had experience with approaching someone with an eating disorder, Jennifer knew that the worst thing to do was to put Amy on the defensive by accusing her, acting judgmental, or making her feel guilty. Jennifer knew that the best approach to take was one of cautious care and concern. Jennifer addressed her concerns about Amy using "I" statements. She told Amy how much she enjoyed training with her and cherished their friendship. She expressed concern about Amy's excessive training and dissatisfaction with her body weight. Jennifer described the struggle her sister went through and worried that perhaps Amy might be having similar problems. She let Amy know that she understood how some people get frustrated with their weight and training and assured Amy that she was there to help her in any way she could. It was a relief for Amy that someone finally understood her and seemed to truly care about her. Amy opened up to Jennifer, telling her about her weight and athletic struggles in college and her unsuccessful counseling sessions. Jennifer convinced Amy to see another psychologist, the same one who had successfully treated her sister.

Three months later, Amy was doing much better. She was meeting regularly with her psychologist and had begun to see a dietitian to develop a healthful eating plan, one that would keep her weight stable and support her training needs. She was finally dealing with the psychological underpinnings of the disorder and was beginning to make progress toward dealing with the factors that precipitated and sustained her addiction to bingeing and purging. For the first time in five years, Amy felt the glimmer of hope. She might be able to get her life back, she might be able to make the Olympic triathlon team, and she had Jennifer to thank for it.

Comment

The course of Amy's bulimia is somewhat unique in terms of the length of time it took to progress. While it certainly can take several years to develop bulimia (as was the case for Amy), generally the clinically significant bulimic behaviors take hold more quickly. Nonetheless, despite the longer progression, the clinical course of Amy's disorder is quite characteristic of athletes who develop bulimia nervosa.

The onset of and the impetus for Amy's weight concerns are typical of athletes who develop bulimia nervosa. As a child and adolescent, Amy was larger than other girls her age, which caused her to become self-conscious about her weight. Her concerns about her weight seemed validated by the chastisement and ridicule that she received regularly from her high school swim coach. This concern led to numerous attempts to shed weight through various dieting methods. As described in chapter 3, individuals who develop bulimia often have a history of overweight or even obesity and of failed dieting attempts. They tend to be very self-conscious about their weight and have low self-esteem. With such fragile body images, it does not take much—a comment or incident concerning weight (such as being called a member of the "fat club") from a person held in high esteem (such as a coach)—to set them into the downward spiral of an eating disorder.

As is true for so many bulimics, Amy turned to food for comfort. Unfortunately, any solace she received from eating was fleeting, as guilt and self-loathing would soon take over. As described in chapter 1, this love–hate relationship is characteristic of those with bulimia nervosa. It is also one of the primary factors leading to and then fueling the binge–purge cycles (as described in chapter 3).

The eating patterns and behaviors that Amy demonstrated during her collegiate swimming career are also characteristic of athletes who develop bulimia nervosa. As described in chapter 1, the athlete usually tries to restrict food intake, to stringently diet, in order to lose weight. Generally the athlete restricts all day only to succumb to hunger and bingeing late at night. Amy's first experience with purging via self-induced vomiting is similar to that described by a number of bulimic athletes. Her first purging experience was not planned but "just happened." Nonetheless, that first purge is like jumping off the high dive for the first time; it is hard to make yourself do it, but it becomes surprisingly easy and ever more frequent as the rush makes you want to do it over and over again. In no time, bulimia becomes almost addictive and takes over the bulimic's life.

The physical and psychological consequences of bulimia (fatigue, sore throat, red and swollen eyes, etc.) experienced by Amy are classic, as was the impetus for her to seek treatment. Indeed, as is so often the case, it took a health crisis to open Amy's eyes and convince her to seek treatment. The failure of initial treatment and subsequent relapse of the bulimic behaviors is unfortunately quite common among individuals diagnosed with eating disorders. Indeed, in many cases, disordered eating is a lifelong disease requiring ongoing treatment.

Often it takes the care and concern of a friend to intervene and break the eating disorder cycle. As described in chapter 10, there is a right way and a wrong way to approach an individual with an eating disorder. Luckily, Amy's friend Jennifer knew the appropriate way to approach her and coax her into seeking treatment.

Case Study 3: Subclinical Eating Disorder

Craig was a high school junior who had been wrestling since he was in junior high school. Up through his freshman year of high school, Craig wrestled in the middle weight class. He was an average wrestler. At the beginning of his sophomore year, Craig's coach suggested that he might do better if he wrestled in a lower weight class. However, because the coach was aware of the sensitivity surrounding weight issues and feared culpability for any consequences Craig might suffer as a result of weight loss, he did not provide Craig with any guidance on how to lose the weight. With only two weeks until the first meet and absolutely no idea how to lose weight, Craig looked in some men's magazines for diet advice. He decided to try a low-carbohydrate, high-protein diet, as it promised that he would lose fat and gain large amounts of muscle. Craig cut out all carbohydrates except a few vegetables and ate large amounts of lean protein (predominantly chicken, turkey, and fish). After one week on the diet, Craig had lost 5 lb (2.3 kg) but was still 5 lb short of the lower weight class (110 lb, or 49.9 kg). In desperation, Craig cut his energy intake in half and increased his training (adding an hour of cardiovascular exercise to his regular wrestling workouts). He just barely made the weight cutoff the day before the meet. Needless to say, the low energy intake combined with the increased training left Craig physically exhausted, and he lost in the first round of the meet.

Craig decided that his poor performance was due to his losing the weight too soon before his meet, so he decided to keep his energy intake low and his energy expenditure high on a regular basis. At the second meet, he did much better, placing second in his weight class. Nonetheless, his chronic energy restriction was taking a toll on him. He was hungry all the time and was chronically fatigued. Craig decided to give himself one "free day" during the week when he could eating anything and everything he wanted. This worked well for a few weeks; he was able to deny himself, knowing that he would have his free day. As the season progressed, however, the time between meets became shorter. Often there were only three or four days between meets, so Craig tried to return to his pattern of chronic energy restriction. After one particularly bad meet, Craig could not stand the hunger and fatigue anymore; he found the nearest convenience store and bought all his favorite (and forbidden) foods—bread, cookies, ice cream, peanut butter—and ate them all at one sitting. Panicked by the knowledge that his next meet was only two days away, he put on sweats and exercised for three hours, followed by two hours in the sauna. He lost the weight quickly, met his weight class, and won the meet. This was the beginning of Craig's bingeing and purging.

As the frequency of binge–purge cycles increased, so too did the difficulty Craig had losing weight. He began to turn to more drastic measures of weight loss, including diuretics and laxatives. He even experimented once or twice with self-induced vomiting, although he did not like to do it and would do so only when nothing else worked.

Craig finished the season well; he was ranked fifth in the state. Over the summer Craig joined a gym and worked out regularly while maintaining a healthful diet. He gave up the low-carbohydrate diet for a diet low in fat with moderate amounts of carbohydrate and protein. He kept his calories down (but not dangerously low) and no longer binged or purged, although occasionally he was tempted to. Craig became very critical of his body shape. He felt that he was soft (although he had only 10% body fat) and longed for the chiseled look of the guys he saw at the gym and in the men's magazines.

When Craig's junior year began, the weight cycling and bingeing and purging began anew. Craig would exercise strenuously and severely restrict his food intake before a meet and binge after the meet was over. Depending on how much time he had to lose weight before the next meet, Craig might or might not use more pathogenic methods of weight loss, such as saunas, a rubber suit, diet pills, laxatives, and occasionally self-induced vomiting.

Comment

Craig does not meet the criteria for either anorexia nervosa or bulimia nervosa. Nonetheless, he does demonstrate disordered eating behaviors. He would likely be classified as having a subclinical eating disorder. As described in chapter 1, those with subclinical eating disorders display similar dieting behaviors and body images as those with the clinical eating disorders anorexia and bulimia nervosa, although with less severity and frequency.

The behaviors displayed by Craig are common among wrestlers (see chapter 4). Craig's pathogenic weight control behaviors were transient, occurring during the season and then subsiding (or disappearing altogether) postseason. Nonetheless, the behaviors and thought processes behind them eventually began to spill over into the off-season. Eventually, Craig began experiencing a degree of body dissatisfaction and guilt surrounding eating that are characteristic of those with subclinical eating disorders (see chapter 1). Moreover, what initially began as a means to an end (i.e., weight loss to make a lower weight class) was becoming an end in itself.

As shown in chapter 3, disordered eating behaviors that are left unchecked can become clinical eating disorders. Thus, it is possible that Craig's disordered eating could progress to a clinical eating disorder, likely bulimia nervosa. As described in chapters 7 and 8, early identification and intervention is the key to reducing the consequences of the disorder and improving treatment outcomes. For Craig, intervention at this point (i.e., early in the development of the eating disorder) is prudent to prevent further health consequences and ensure a more favorable outcome.

Disordered Eating Assessment

Assessment Parameters for Disordered Eating Screening

The following list outlines the physical and psychological parameters that should be assessed when screening for disordered eating among athletes.

1. Weight
   - Highest
   - Lowest
   - Perceived ideal
2. Body image
   - Degree of satisfaction with overall weight and shape
   - Degree of satisfaction with specific body parts
3. Nutritional history
   - Food log (at least three days) to assess usual intake
   - Number of meals and snacks per day
   - Frequency of skipped meals
   - Nutritional beliefs and practices (e.g., vegetarian?)
4. Methods of weight control
   - Calorie restriction (ascertain a calorie level)
   - Avoidance of particular foods (ascertain which foods)
   - Bingeing
     - Frequency
     - Time of day or night
     - Amount of food consumed
   - Purging
     - Vomiting
     - Laxatives

- Diuretics
- Diet pills
- Excessive exercise

5. Exercise history
   - Sport participation
   - Hours spent training per week
   - Time spent exercising outside of normal training or practice for sport

6. Menstrual history
   - Age of menarche
   - Frequency and duration of periods
   - Number of times periods have been missed (amenorrhea)
   - Date of last menstrual period
   - Use of oral contraceptives or hormonal therapy

7. Physical or laboratory exam
   - Physical signs and symptoms of starvation (see later section in this appendix)
   - Physical signs and symptoms of bingeing and purging (see later section in this appendix)
   - Biochemical measures
     - Electrolytes
     - Blood urea nitrogen (BUN)
     - Creatinine
     - Liver function
     - Amylase
     - Calcium, phosphorous, magnesium
     - Iron
     - Thyroid function

Physical Signs and Symptoms of Eating Disorders

The following list outlines the physical signs and symptoms associated with anorexia and bulimia nervosa.

Anorexia Nervosa
- Bradycardia
- Orthostatic hypotension (by pulse or blood pressure)
- Hypothermia
- Cardiac murmur (mitral valve prolapse)

- Dull, thinning hair
- Sunken cheeks, sallow skin
- Lanugo
- Atrophic breasts (postpubertal)
- Pitting edema of extremities
- Cold extremities
- Parotid gland enlargement
- Gastrointestinal complaints

Bulimia Nervosa
- Sinus bradycardia
- Orthostatic hypotension (by pulse or blood pressure)
- Hypothermia
- Cardiac arrhythmia
- Dull hair
- Dry skin
- Parotitis
- Russell's sign (calluses on knuckles from self-induced vomiting)
- Mouth sores
- Palatal scratches
- Dental enamel erosion
- Sore, irritated throat
- Gastrointestinal complaints

Laboratory and Biochemical Findings Associated With Eating Disorders

The following list outlines the alternatives in biochemical indicies frequently seen with anorexia and bulimia nervosa.

Anorexia Nervosa
- Decreased iron status measures (anemia is common)
- Elevation of liver enzymes
- Hypoglycemia
- Decreased serum creatinine
- Decreased BUN
- Low thyroid function (decreased T4)
- Hypophosphatemia
- Hypocholesterolemia (low HDL and LDL levels)

Bulimia Nervosa

- Decreased iron status measures (anemia is common)
- Hyponatremia
- Hypokalemia
- Metabolic alkalosis (associated with self-induced vomiting)
- Metabolic acidosis (associated with laxative abuse; may mask a potassium deficiency)
- Hypomagnesemia
- Hypoglycemia (due to purging)
- Hyperglycemia (due to bingeing)
- Dehydration

appendix C
Educational Resources

Books

Sports Nutrition

Berning, J.R., ed. 2002. *Sports nutrition patient education resource manual*. Rockville, MD: Aspen Publishers, Inc.

Burke, L., and V. Deakin, eds. 2002. *Clinical sports nutrition*. New York, NY: McGraw Hill.

Clark, N. 2003. *Sports nutrition guidebook 3rd edition*. Champaign, IL: Human Kinetics.

Dorfman, L. 1999. *The vegetarian sports nutrition guide: Peak performance for everyone from beginners to gold medalists*. New York, NY: John Wiley and Sons.

Manore, M.M. and J. Thompson. 2000. *Sport nutrition for health and performance*. Champaign, IL: Human Kinetics.

Rosenbloom, C.A. 1999. *Sports nutrition: A guide for the professional working with active people. 3rd ed.* Chicago, IL: American Dietetic Association.

Wolinsky, I., and J.A. Driskell, eds. 2001. *Nutritional applications in exercise and sport*. Boca Raton, FL: CRC Press.

Eating Disorder

Andersen, A.E., and P.S. Mehler, eds. 1999. Eating disorders: A guide to medical care and complications. Baltimore, MD: John's Hopkins University Press.

Claude-Pierre, P. 1998. The secrete language of eating disorders: How you can understand and work to cure anorexia and bulimia. UK: Vintage.

Costin, C. 1999. The eating disorder sourcebook: A comprehensive guide to causes, treatments and prevention. New York, NY: McGraw Hill.

Otis, C. and R. Goldingay. 2000. The athletic woman's survival guide. How to win the battle against eating disorders, amenorrhea and osteoporosis. Champaign, IL: Human Kinetics.

Thompson, J.K., ed. 1996. Body image, Eating disorders, and obesity: An integrated guide for assessment and treatment. Washington, DC: American Psychological Association.

Web Sites

Eating Disorders

About Face   www.about-face.org

Academy for Eating Disorders (AED)   www.aedweb.org

American Anorexia and Bulimia Society (AABA)   www.members.aol.com/amanbu.org

American Psychiatric Association   www.psych.org

American Psychological Association   www.apa.org

Anorexia Nervosa and Related Eating Disorders, Inc.   www.anred.com

Body Positive   www.bodypositive.com

Center for Change   www.centerforchange.com

Council on Size and Weight Discrimination   www.cswd.org

Eating Disorder Referral and Information Center   www.edreferral.com

Eating Disorders Anonymous   www.eatingdisordersanonymous.org

Eating Disorders Awareness and Prevention, Inc.   http://members.aol.com/edapinc/home.html

Eating Disorders Information   http://members.tripod.com/~rfehr/Ed2.htm

Harvard Eating Disorders Center   www.hedc.org

International Association of Eating Disorders Professionals   www.iaedp.com

Massachusetts Eating Disorder Association, Inc. (MEDA)   www.medainc.org

National Association of Anorexia Nervosa and Associated Disorders   www.anad.org

National Eating Disorder Information Center   www.bedic

National Eating Disorders Association   www.nationaleatingdisorders.org

National Eating Disorder Screening Program   www.mentalhealthscreening.org/eat.htm

NCAA CHAMPS Life Skills Program   www1.ncaa.org/membership/ed_outreach/champs-life_skills/index.html

NCAA Educational Resources   www.ncaa.org/sports_sciences/education

Ohio State University   http://ohiostatebuckeyes.ocsn.com/genrel/sa-handbook/conduct.PDF

Overeaters Anonymous (OA)   www.nmisp.org

Renfrew Center Foundation   www.renfrew.org

Something Fishy   www.something-fishy.org

Vitality Inc.: Promoting Wellness and Respect for All Shapes   www.tiac.net/users/vtlty

Westwind Eating Disorder Recovery Centre   www.westwtnd.mb.ca

Nutrition

American College of Sportsmedicine   www.acsm.org

American Dietetic Association   www.eatright.org

Federal Government Information on Nutrition   www.nutrition.gov

Gatorade Sports Science Institute   www.gssiweb.com

Sports, Cardiovascular and Wellness Nutritionists   www.scandpg.org

CSPI- The Center for Science in the Public Interest   www.cspinet.org

Nutrition Quackery Watchdog   www.quackwatch.com

appendix D

High-Carbohydrate, Lower-Fat Food Choices

Foods	Amount	Carbohydrate (g)	Fat (g)
Bread, rice, pasta, and legumes			
Angel food cake	1 slice (53 g)	32	<1
Bagel	1 (55 g)	38	1
Bran muffin	1 (40 g)	25	<1
Bun	1 (42 g)	22	2
English muffin	1 (56 g)	26	1
Garbanzo beans	1/2 c (130 g)	18	1
Kidney beans	1/2 c (130 g)	19	1
Pancake or waffle	1 (27 g)	15	2
Pasta	1/2 c (70 g)	16	0
Pita bread	1 slice (38 g)	33	1
Popcorn (plain)	1 c (25 g)	4	<1
Pretzels	1 oz (28 g)	19	<1
Rice, brown (cooked)	1/2 c (97.5 g)	23	1
Rice, white (cooked)	1/2 c (72 g)	17	<1
Rice cake	1 (9 g)	8	<1
Tortilla (flour)	1 (10 in., or 25 cm)	40	4
Whole wheat bread	1 slice (28 g)	13	1
Cereals (low in refined sugar)			
Bran flakes	1 c (37 g)	24	<1
Cheerios	1 c (23 g)	17	1.5
Grape-Nuts	1/2 c (54.5 g)	45	<1
Oatmeal (cooked)	1 c (234 g)	25	3
Shredded wheat	1 biscuit (24 g)	19	<1

(continued)

Foods	Amount	Carbohydrate (g)	Fat (g)
Crackers			
Graham	1 (7 g)	5	<1
Rye Krisp	1 (7 g)	5	<1
Saltine	1 (3 g)	2	<1
Vegetables			
Carrots	1/2 c (78 g)	8	0
Corn	1/2 c (82 g)	16	0
Peas (sweet)	1/2 c (80 g)	11	0
Potato (white)	1 medium (122 g)	29	0
Sweet potato	1 medium (121 g)	28	0
Tomato (fresh)	1/2 c (90 g)	4	0
Tomato juice	1/2 c (118 ml)	5	0
Fruits			
Apple (dried)	1/4 c (21.5 g)	14	0
Apple (whole)	1 medium (160 g)	21	<1
Apple juice	3/4 c (177 ml)	22	0
Apricot (dried)	1/4 c (32.5 g)	20	0
Banana (whole)	1 medium (118 g)	28	<1
Cantaloupe	1/2 c (80 g)	7	0
Cranberry juice	3/4 c (177 ml)	27	0
Fig (whole)	1 medium (50 g)	10	0
Grape juice	3/4 c (177 ml)	24	0
Grapes	1/2 c (80 g)	14	0
Orange (whole)	1 medium (131 g)	15	0
Orange juice	3/4 c (177 ml)	19	0
Peach (whole)	1 medium (98 g)	11	0
Peaches (canned)	1/2 c (122 g)	8	0
Pear (whole)	1 medium (166 g)	25	<1
Pears (canned)	1/2 c (124 g)	16	0
Pineapple (canned)	1/2 c (77.5 g)	10	0
Raisins	1/4 c (41 g)	32	0
Watermelon	1/2 c (76 g)	6	0
Milk products			
Milk, 1%	1 c (237 ml)	12	2.5

Foods	Amount	Carbohydrate (g)	Fat (g)
Milk, 1% chocolate	1 c (237 ml)	26	2.5
Milk, skim	1 c (237 ml)	12	0
Pudding (nonfat)	1/2 c (118 ml)	23	0
Yogurt (low-fat)	1 c (237 ml)	17	3
Yogurt (nonfat)	1 c (237 ml)	43	<1
Yogurt, frozen (low-fat)	1/2 c (118 ml)	21	2
Yogurt, frozen (nonfat)	1/2 c (118 ml)	21	<1
Combination foods			
Bean burrito	1 small	50	10
Macaroni and cheese	1/2 c (98 g)	24	8
Pasta with tomato sauce	1 c (166 g)	36	3
Pizza, veggie	1 slice	29	10
Potato salad	1/2 c (125 g)	14	10
Taco, meat	1	27	9
Tomato soup	1 c (237 ml)	17	2
Turkey sandwich	1 (6 in., or 15 cm)	46	3
Vegetable lasagna	1 piece (156 g)	17	10
Vegetable sandwich	1 (6 in., or 15 cm)	44	3
Vegetable soup	1 c (237 ml)	12	2
Sweets			

Candy
    Hard candy
    Gum drops
	
	1 oz (28 g)
	1 oz (28 g)
		
		28
		25
			
			0
			0

Cookies
    Fig bar
    Granola bar (low fat)
    Oatmeal raisin
    Snackwell's cookies
	
	1 (26 g)
	1 (14 g)
	9 (42 g)
	2 (28 g)
		
		19
		11
		32
		32
			
			4
			<1
			2.5
			3

Jam or jelly	1 Tbsp (15 ml)	13	0
Juice drink	1 c (237 ml)	41	0
Maple syrup	1 Tbsp (15 ml)	14	0
Soft drinks	1 c (237 ml)	25	0
Commercial sports drinks and foods			
Clif Bar	1 (68 g)	51	4
Gatorade	1 c (237 ml)	15	0

(continued)

Foods	Amount	Carbohydrate (g)	Fat (g)
GatorLode	1 c (237 ml)	47	0
GatorPro	1 c (237 ml)	58	0
Luna bar	1 (48 g)	26	4.5
Nutrament	1 c (237 ml)	30	0
Powerade	1 c (237 ml)	19	0
PowerBar	1 (63 g)	40	0
Ultra Fuel	1 c (237 ml)	50	0

Eating Disorder Screening Questionnaires

Eating Attitudes Test

The Eating Attitudes Test (EAT-26) is probably the most widely used standardized measure of symptoms and characteristics of eating disorders. The EAT-26 alone does not yield a specific diagnosis of an eating disorder. Neither the EAT-26 nor any other screening instrument has been established as highly efficient as the sole means for identifying eating disorders. However, studies have shown that the EAT-26 can be an efficient screening instrument as part of a two-stage screening process in which those who score at or above a cutoff score of 20 are referred for a diagnostic interview.

	1 Always	2 Very often	3 Often	4 Sometimes	5 Rarely	6 Never
1. I am terrified about being overweight.	1	2	3	4	5	6
2. I avoid eating when I am hungry.	1	2	3	4	5	6
3. I find myself preoccupied with food.	1	2	3	4	5	6
4. I have gone on eating binges where I feel that I may not be able to stop.	1	2	3	4	5	6

(continued)

	1 Always	2 Very often	3 Often	4 Sometimes	5 Rarely	6 Never
5. I cut my food into small pieces.	1	2	3	4	5	6
6. I am aware of the calorie content of foods that I eat.	1	2	3	4	5	6
7. I particularly avoid foods with high carbohydrate content.	1	2	3	4	5	6
8. I feel that others would prefer if I ate more.	1	2	3	4	5	6
9. I vomit after I have eaten.	1	2	3	4	5	6
10. I feel extremely guilty after eating.	1	2	3	4	5	6
11. I am preoccupied with a desire to be thinner.	1	2	3	4	5	6
12. I think about burning up calories when I exercise.	1	2	3	4	5	6
13. Other people think I am too thin.	1	2	3	4	5	6
14. I am preoccupied with the thought of having fat on my body.	1	2	3	4	5	6
15. I take longer than others to eat meals.	1	2	3	4	5	6
16. I avoid foods with sugar in them.	1	2	3	4	5	6

	1 Always	2 Very often	3 Often	4 Sometimes	5 Rarely	6 Never
17. I eat diet foods.	1	2	3	4	5	6
18. I feel that food controls my life.	1	2	3	4	5	6
19. I display self-control around food.	1	2	3	4	5	6
20. I feel that others pressure me to eat.	1	2	3	4	5	6
21. I give too much time and thought to food.	1	2	3	4	5	6
22. I feel uncomfortable after eating sweets.	1	2	3	4	5	6
23. I engage in dieting behavior.	1	2	3	4	5	6
24. I like my stomach to be empty.	1	2	3	4	5	6
25. I enjoy trying new rich foods.	1	2	3	4	5	6
26. I have the impulse to vomit after meals.	1	2	3	4	5	6

From D. M. Garner et al, 1982, "The eating attitudes test: psychometric features and clinical correlates," *Psychological Medicine* 12: 871-878. Reprinted with the permission of Cambridge University Press.

Scoring for the EAT-26

The response for each of the 26 items is given a score from 0 to 3; a score of 3 is assigned to the responses farthest in the symptomatic direction, a score of 2 for the immediately adjacent response, a score of 1 for the next adjacent response, and a score of 0 for the three responses farthest in the asymptomatic direction. Note that question 25 is scored in reverse; that is, the symptomatic direction is opposite that of the other items.

Eating Disorder Inventory

The Eating Disorder Inventory (EDI) is a screening instrument frequently used in both research and clinical settings. The EDI measures the psychological and behavioral traits common in anorexia nervosa and bulimia nervosa. The EDI contains eight different constructs or subscales, including (1) Drive for Thinness, (2) Bulimia, (3) Body Dissatisfaction, (4) Ineffectiveness, (5) Perfectionism, (6) Interpersonal Distrust, (7) Interoceptive Awareness, and (8) Maturity Fears.

	1 Always	2 Very often	3 Often	4 Sometimes	5 Rarely	6 Never
1. I eat sweets and carbohydrates without feeling guilty.	1	2	3	4	5	6
2. I get frightened when my feelings are too strong.	1	2	3	4	5	6
3. I think about dieting.	1	2	3	4	5	6
4. I get confused about what emotion I am feeling.	1	2	3	4	5	6
5. I eat when I am upset.	1	2	3	4	5	6
6. I think that my stomach is too big.	1	2	3	4	5	6
7. I feel ineffective as a person.	1	2	3	4	5	6
8. I wish that I could return to the security of childhood.	1	2	3	4	5	6
9. Only an outstanding performance is good enough in my family.	1	2	3	4	5	6
10. I am open about my feelings.	1	2	3	4	5	6
11. I stuff myself with food.	1	2	3	4	5	6

	1 Always	2 Very often	3 Often	4 Sometimes	5 Rarely	6 Never
12. I think that my thighs are too large.	1	2	3	4	5	6
13. I feel alone in the world.	1	2	3	4	5	6
14. I wish that I could be younger.	1	2	3	4	5	6
15. As a child, I tried very hard to avoid disappointing my parents.	1	2	3	4	5	6
16. I trust others.	1	2	3	4	5	6
17. I feel extremely guilty after overeating.	1	2	3	4	5	6
18. I can clearly identify what emotion I'm feeling.	1	2	3	4	5	6
19. I have gone on eating binges where I have felt that I could not stop.	1	2	3	4	5	6
20. I think that my stomach is just the right size.	1	2	3	4	5	6
21. I feel generally in control of things in my life.	1	2	3	4	5	6
22. The happiest time in life is when you are a child.	1	2	3	4	5	6
23. I hate being less than the best at things.	1	2	3	4	5	6

(continued)

	1 Always	2 Very often	3 Often	4 Sometimes	5 Rarely	6 Never
24. I can communi-cate with others easily.	1	2	3	4	5	6
25. I am terrified of gaining weight.	1	2	3	4	5	6
26. I don't know what's going on inside of me.	1	2	3	4	5	6
27. I think about overeating.	1	2	3	4	5	6
28. I feel satisfied with the shape of my body.	1	2	3	4	5	6
29. I wish I were someone else.	1	2	3	4	5	6
30. I would rather be an adult than a child.	1	2	3	4	5	6
31. My parents have expected excel-lence of me.	1	2	3	4	5	6
32. I have close relationships.	1	2	3	4	5	6
33. I exaggerate or magnify the importance of weight.	1	2	3	4	5	6
34. I get confused as to whether or not I am hungry.	1	2	3	4	5	6
35. I eat moderately in front of others and stuff myself when I am alone.	1	2	3	4	5	6
36. I like the shape of my buttocks.	1	2	3	4	5	6
37. I feel inad-equate.	1	2	3	4	5	6

	1 Always	2 Very often	3 Often	4 Sometimes	5 Rarely	6 Never
38. The demands of adulthood are too great.	1	2	3	4	5	6
39. I feel that I must do things perfectly or not do them at all.	1	2	3	4	5	6
40. I have trouble expressing my emotions to others.	1	2	3	4	5	6
41. I am preoccupied with the desire to be thinner.	1	2	3	4	5	6
42. I worry that my feelings will get out of control.	1	2	3	4	5	6
43. I have thought of trying to vomit in order to lose weight.	1	2	3	4	5	6
44. I think my hips are too big.	1	2	3	4	5	6
45. I feel secure about myself.	1	2	3	4	5	6
46. I feel that people are happiest when they are children.	1	2	3	4	5	6
47. I have extremely high goals.	1	2	3	4	5	6
48. I feel happy that I am not a child anymore.	1	2	3	4	5	6
49. If I gain a pound I worry that I will keep gaining.	1	2	3	4	5	6

(continued)

	1 Always	2 Very often	3 Often	4 Sometimes	5 Rarely	6 Never
50. I feel bloated after eating a small meal.	1	2	3	4	5	6
51. When I am upset I don't know if I am sad, frightened, or angry.	1	2	3	4	5	6
52. I eat or drink in secrecy.	1	2	3	4	5	6
53. I think my thighs are just the right size.	1	2	3	4	5	6
54. I have a low opinion of myself.	1	2	3	4	5	6
55. The best years of your life are when you become an adult.	1	2	3	4	5	6
56. I feel that I can achieve my standards.	1	2	3	4	5	6
57. I need to keep people at a certain distance (feel uncomfortable if someone tries to get too close).	1	2	3	4	5	6
58. I think my buttocks are too large.	1	2	3	4	5	6
59. I feel that I am a worthwhile person.	1	2	3	4	5	6
60. I have feelings I can't quite identify.	1	2	3	4	5	6

	1 Always	2 Very often	3 Often	4 Sometimes	5 Rarely	6 Never
61. When I am upset I worry that I will start to eat.	1	2	3	4	5	6
62. I think that my hips are just the right size.	1	2	3	4	5	6
63. I feel emotionally empty inside.	1	2	3	4	5	6
64. I can talk about personal thoughts or feelings.	1	2	3	4	5	6

Reprinted, by permission, from D.M. Garner, M.P. Olmstead and J. Polivy, 1983, "Development and validation of a multidimensional eating disorder inventory for anorexia nervosa and bulimia," *International Journal of Eating Disorders* 2(2):15-34.

Scoring for the EDI

The response for each item is given a score from 0 to 3, with a score of 3 assigned to the response farthest in the symptomatic direction, a score of 2 for the immediately adjacent response, a score of 1 for the next adjacent response, and a score of 0 for the three responses farthest in the asymptomatic direction. Questions 1, 10, 16, 18, 20, 21, 24, 28, 32, 36, 45, 53, 55, 56, 59, 62, and 64 are scored in reverse.

- Drive for Thinness subscale: questions 1, 3, 17, 25, 33, 41, 49
- Bulimia subscale: questions 5, 11, 19, 27, 35, 43, 52
- Body Dissatisfaction subscale: questions 6, 12, 20, 28, 36, 44, 53, 58, 62
- Ineffectiveness subscale: questions 7, 13, 21, 29, 37, 45, 54, 56, 59, 63
- Perfectionism subscale: questions 9, 15, 23, 31, 39, 47
- Interpersonal Distrust subscale: questions 10, 16, 24, 32, 40, 57, 64
- Interoceptive Awareness subscale: questions 2, 4, 18, 26, 34, 42, 50, 51, 60, 61
- Maturity Fears subscale: questions 8, 14, 22, 30, 38, 46, 48, 55

Sample Preparticipation Screening Instruments

Ball State University
Student-Athlete Health Questionnaire

This questionnaire was developed as part of an ongoing research study designed to assess the prevalence of disordered eating and menstrual dysfunction among collegiate athletes.

Demographic Information

1. Primary sport you participate in: _____

2. Birth date (mo/d/yr): _____

3. Years of participation in your sport: lifetime: _____ collegiate: _____

4. Age: _____

5. Ethnicity (check one):
   ___ African American ___ Asian ___ Caucasian
   ___ Hispanic ___ other (describe)

6. Year in school (check one):
   ___ Freshman ___ Sophomore ___ Junior ___ Senior ___ Graduate

Gynecological/Menstrual History

7. Have you ever had a menstrual period? ___ yes ___ no (skip to #18)

8. How old were you when you had your first menstrual period? _____

9. How many menstrual periods have you had in the last 12 months? _____

10. How many days are there between your periods? _____

11. How many days do your periods (bleeding) last? _____

12. How would you describe your menstrual bleeding?
    ___ light ___ moderate ___ heavy

13. Use your response to question #10 to determine the regularity of your cycle (check one):

___ I am very regular (within 3 days)

___ I am somewhat irregular (4-10 day variation)

___ I am very irregular (variation greater than 10 days)

14. When was your last period (mo/yr)? _____

15. Do your periods change with changes in your training regimen?

___ yes ___ no

  • If yes, please describe how they change: _____

_____

16. Have you ever gone for more than 3 months without having a menstrual period? ___ yes ___ no

  • If yes: How old were you when you first missed ≥3 periods? _____

  • How long did you go without menstruating? (months) _____

  • How many times have you gone for more than 3 months without having a period? _____

17. Do you currently take birth control pills? ___ yes ___ no

  • If yes: What are you using them for?

    ___ birth control ___ regulate menstrual cycle ___ both

  • How long have you been using birth control pills? (months) _____

18. Have you had a pelvic exam? ___ yes ___ no

Date of last exam (mo/yr): _____

19. Please describe any other menstrual irregularities or problems not already covered in the above questions. _____

_____

Musculoskeletal History

20. Is your frame size: ___ small ___ medium ___ large

21. Is there a history of osteoporosis in your family? ___ yes ___ no

22. Have you ever sustained a stress fracture? ___ yes ___ no

  • If yes, describe the injury site(s)   date(s) the injury/injuries was/were sustained:

    _____   _____

    _____   _____

    _____   _____

23. Have you sustained any other musculoskeletal injuries within the past year? ___ yes ___ no

  • If yes, describe the injury/injuries and date(s) sustained _____

_____

Weight History

24. Height: _____
25. Weight: _____
26. Length of time at current weight (months): _____
27. How many times has your weight fluctuated by at least 5 lb in the last year? _____
28. What is your "ideal" weight? _____
29. When (age) were you last at your ideal weight? _____
30. Do you consciously control your weight for your sport?

    ___ yes ___ no • If you did not consciously control your weight, what do you think it would be? _____
31. When your season is over and you stop or reduce your training, do you

    ___ gain weight (amount: _____)

    ___ lose weight (amount: _____) ___ maintain weight
32. How often are you dieting *during the season?*

    ___ never ___ rarely ___ sometimes ___ often ___ always
33. How often are you dieting *during the off-season or when you stop or reduce training?* ___ never ___ rarely ___ sometimes ___ often ___ always
34. Over the past year have you used any of the following methods to control your weight? • Please indicate yes or no and, if yes, the number of times you used that method.

Method	Yes	No	# of times used
Commercial weight loss programs (e.g., Jenny Craig, Weight Watchers)			
Over-the-counter diet pills (e.g., Dexatrim)			
Fasting			
Liquid diet supplements (e.g., Slim-Fast)			
Very low calories (< 800 kcal/d)			
Laxatives			
Diuretics			
Vomiting			
Skipping meals			
High protein, low carbohydrate			
Nutritional counseling with a health care professional (dietitian)			
Additional exercise beyond regular training			
Other (please describe)			

35. Which of the following are you currently trying to do about your weight?

    ___ lose weight ___ gain weight ___ stay the same weight

36. What percentage of your exercise is aimed at weight control?

    ___ 0% ___ ≤ 25% ___ 26%-50% ___ 51%-75% ___ 76%-100%

37. I presently think of myself as being

    ___ very underweight (>10 lb)

    ___ slightly underweight (5-10 lb)

    ___ at an "ideal" weight

    ___ slightly overweight (<10 lb)

    ___ moderately overweight (10-20 lb)

    ___ very overweight (>20 lb)

38. Other people say that I am presently

    ___ very underweight (>10 lb)

    ___ slightly underweight (5-10 lb)

    ___ at an "ideal" weight

    ___ slightly overweight (<10 lb)

    ___ moderately overweight (10-20 lb)

    ___ very overweight (>20 lb)

39. Do you feel pressure to achieve or maintain a particular body weight?

    ___ yes ___ no

    • If yes, from whom do you feel pressure? (check all that apply)

      ___ myself ___ parents ___ teammates ___ society ___ coach

      ___ trainers ___ boyfriend/partner ___ friends

40. How satisfied are you with your body weight?

    ___ very satisfied ___ satisfied ___ neutral

    ___ dissatisfied ___ very dissatisfied

41. How satisfied are you with your current body size or shape?

    ___ very satisfied ___ satisfied ___ neutral

    ___ dissatisfied ___ very dissatisfied

Nutrition History

42. How many meals (i.e., breakfast, lunch, dinner) do you usually eat per day? (check one)

    ___ 1-2 ___ 3-4 ___ 5-6 ___ more than 6

43. How many snacks do you usually eat per day? (check one)

    ___ 1-2 ___ 3-4 ___ 5-6 ___ more than 6

44. Do you skip meals?

    ___ never ___ rarely ___ sometimes ___ often ___ always

45. Please check any of the following food groups that you avoid (check all that apply):

___ red meat   ___ breads and grains (pasta, rice)

___ poultry (chicken, turkey)   ___ eggs

___ fish   ___ fast foods

___ dairy (milk, cheese)   ___ sweets (candy, desserts)

___ vegetables   ___ fried foods

___ fruits

___ fats or oils (mayonnaise, salad dressings, butter)

46. Please check the average number of dairy (milk, yogurt, cheese) products you typically eat:

___ 0 ___ 3-4 per week ___ 1-2 per day ___ 1-2 per week

___ 5-6 per week ___ 3-4 per day

47. Do you think your diet is nutritionally adequate? ___ yes ___ no

48. Do you drink alcohol? ___ yes ___ no

• If yes, indicate the amount per week: _____

49. Do you smoke? ___ yes ___ no

• If yes, indicate number of cigarettes per day: _____

50. Do you take vitamin or mineral supplements?

___ yes, daily ___ yes, but not every day ___ no (skip to #52)

51. Please indicate the type(s) of supplement(s) you use (check all that apply):

___ multivitamin   ___ multivitamin/mineral   ___ iron

___ zinc   ___ vitamin C   ___ magnesium

___ vitamin E   ___ B-complex vitamins   ___ calcium

___ chromium

___ other (please describe): _____

52. Do you use nutritional supplements or sports products?

___ yes, daily ___ yes, but not every day ___ no (skip to #54)

53. Please indicate the type(s) of supplement(s) you use (check all that apply):

___ protein powder/drink   ___ sports bars (PowerBar, Clif Bar)

___ amino acids   ___ sports drinks (Gatorade, Powerade)

___ HMB   ___ "fat burners" (ephedrine, ma huang)

___ glutamine   ___ pyruvate

___ creatine   ___ hormones (androstenedione, DHEA)

___ other (please describe): _____

54. Do you ever feel out of control when eating or feel that you cannot stop eating? ___ yes ___ no

55. Have you ever eaten a large amount of food rapidly (i.e., binged) and felt that this eating incident was excessive and out of control (aside from holiday feasts)? ___ yes ___ no
   - If yes, how often have you engaged in this behavior during the past year?
     ___ ≤ once a month ___ 2-3 times per month ___ ≤ once a week
     ___ > once a week ___ daily

56. How many times have you binged (eaten >1,200 kcal at a single sitting) in the past month? _____

57. Have you ever purged after a binge? ___ yes ___ no
   - If yes, what type of purging did you engage in? (check all that apply)
     ___ laxatives ___ vomiting ___ diuretics ___ excessive exercise

58. Do you think you might have an eating disorder?
   ___ yes ___ no ___ maybe

59. Have you ever been clinically diagnosed or treated for anorexia nervosa? ___ yes ___ no
   - If yes, please indicate
     age at diagnosis: _____
     length of time the eating disorder lasted: _____

60. Have you ever been clinically diagnosed or treated for bulimia nervosa? ___ yes ___ no
   - If yes, please indicate
     age at diagnosis: _____
     length of time the eating disorder lasted: _____

From Ball State University Student Athlete Health/ Nutrition Survey, 2002. Reprinted by permission of K. Beals.

University of Utah
Freshman Athlete Health Screen

The screening instrument used by the University of Utah is administered to all incoming freshman female athletes.

Date: _____

Personal Information

Name: _____ Sport: _____
Position: _____ Years in sport: _____
School year: _____ Age: _____ DOB: _____
Address: _____
Phone: _____ Hometown: _____

Training Schedule

Training begins: _____ Competition begins: _____
Weekly training schedule (strength/cond/skills)

Outside training:

Medical Information

Last physical exam date: _____
Results: _____
Medications: _____
Allergies (food/med): _____
Limitations/injuries (medical problems):

_____

Hospitalizations/surgeries:

_____

Broken bones/stress fractures:

_____

General Health

Concentration: _____ Fatigue: _____
Irritability/anxiousness: _____
GI distress (diarrhea, constipation, vomiting):

_____

Sleep disturbance:
    Too much/Too little   Trouble falling asleep
Depression: _____

(continued)

Menstrual History

Age at start menses: _____   # Periods past 12 months: _____

Periods are: regular   irregular   absent   Last period date: _____

Birth control pills/Depo-Provera?

_____

Current or last 12 months _____

Periods change with training/season?   Yes   No

Weight History

Current Ht: _____ Wt: _____   When measured:_____

How often: _____   Usual Wt:_____   "Ideal"Wt: _____

Highest Wt: _____   When/how long: _____

Lowest Wt: _____   When/how long: _____

Weight change with training/season?   Yes   No

Tried to control weight?   Yes   No   How?_____

_____

Weight control methods (list frequency):

Diet pills _____   Current   Past

Diuretics _____   Current   Past

Vomiting_____   Current   Past

Fasting _____   Current   Past

Laxatives_____   Current   Past

Exercise_____   Current   Past

Special Diet _____   Current   Past

Other: _____

Diet History

Meals/day: _____ Snacks/day: _____ Eating-out frequency: _____

Vit/Min supplements: _____

Other supplements:_____

Food frequency *(per day/wk/mo):*

Red meat: _____   Bread:_____

Poultry: _____   Cereal: _____

Fish: _____   Rice: _____

Eggs: _____   Pasta: _____

Beans/lentils: _____   Potatoes: _____

Milk: _____   Fats: _____

Yogurt:_____   Fried foods: _____

Cheese: _____   Peanut butter/nuts: _____
Vegetables: _____   Candy: _____
Fruit: _____   Desserts: _____
Juice: _____   Coffee/Tea: _____
Soda (type): _____   Alcohol: _____
Water: _____   Avoid fat? _____
Forbidden foods: _____

Typical daily intake:

Time	Food	Amount
_____	_____	_____
_____	_____	_____
_____	_____	_____
_____	_____	_____
_____	_____	_____
_____	_____	_____
_____	_____	_____
_____	_____	_____
_____	_____	_____
_____	_____	_____
_____	_____	_____

Summary

Evidence of disordered eating: Yes No _____
Evidence of depression: Yes No _____
Problems/concerns: _____
_____
Recommendations: _____
_____
Referrals: _____
_____
Notes: _____
_____
_____
Follow-up: Yes No _____
_____

Signature:
_____

Annual Screen

UCLA Sports Medicine
Preparticipation Exam

❏ New
❏ Returning

The following screening instrument is used to identify disordered eating in UCLA athletes.

Name _____ Date of Exam _____

Sport _____ Sex: (M) ❏ (F) ❏ Age _____ DOB _____

Campus Address _____

Explain "Yes" answers below.

Circle questions you don't know the answers to   **YES   NO**

1. Have you ever had a medical illness or injury since your last check-up or sports physical?   ❏   ❏

   Do you have any ongoing or chronic illness?   ❏   ❏

   Have you ever been hospitalized overnight?   ❏   ❏

2. Have you ever had surgery?   ❏   ❏

3. Have you ever had a sprain, strain, or swelling after injury?   ❏   ❏

   Have you broken or fractured any bones or dislocated any joints?   ❏   ❏

   Have you had any other problems with pain or swelling in muscles, tendons, bones, or joints?   ❏   ❏

   If yes, check appropriate box and explain below.

   ❏ Head   ❏ Elbow   ❏ Thigh
   ❏ Neck   ❏ Forearm   ❏ Knee
   ❏ Back   ❏ Wrist   ❏ Shin/Calf
   ❏ Chest   ❏ Hand   ❏ Ankle
   ❏ Shoulder   ❏ Finger   ❏ Foot
   ❏ Upper arm   ❏ Hip

4. Are you currently taking any prescriptions (including female hormones/oral contraceptives) or non-prescription (over-the-counter) medications, pills or using an inhaler?   ❏   ❏

   Do you have allergies to *any* medications?   ❏   ❏

   Have you ever taken any supplements or vitamins to help you gain or lose weight or improve your performance?   ❏   ❏

5. Do you have a broken, chipped or loose tooth or dental plate?   ❏   ❏

	YES	NO

6. Has a physician ever denied or restricted your participation in sports for any heart problems? ❏ ❏

Have you ever passed out during or after exercise? ❏ ❏

Have you ever been dizzy during or after exercise? ❏ ❏

Have you ever had chest pain during or after exercise? ❏ ❏

Do you get tired more quickly than your friends do during exercise? ❏ ❏

Have you ever had racing of the heart or had your heart skip heartbeats? ❏ ❏

Have you ever had high blood pressure or high cholesterol? ❏ ❏

Have you had any tests for your heart? ❏ ❏

Have you ever been told you have a heart murmur? ❏ ❏

Has any family member or relative died of heart problems or died suddenly before the age of 50? ❏ ❏

Have you had a severe viral infection (for example myocarditis or mononucleosis) within the last month? ❏ ❏

7. Are you missing one of the following: kidney, eye, testicle (or an undescended testicle)? ❏ ❏

8. Do you have any current skin problems (for example, itching, rashes, acne, warts, fungus, or blisters)? ❏ ❏

9. Have you ever had a head injury or concussion? ❏ ❏

Have you ever been knocked-out, become unconscious or lost your memory? ❏ ❏

Have you ever had a seizure? ❏ ❏

Do you have frequent or severe headaches? ❏ ❏

Have you ever had numbness or tingling in your arms, hands, legs, or feet? ❏ ❏

Have you ever had a stinger, burner, or pinched nerve? ❏ ❏

10. Have you ever become ill from exercising in the heat? ❏ ❏

11. Do you cough, wheeze, or have trouble breathing during or after activity or have asthma? ❏ ❏

Have you ever developed hives with exercise? ❏ ❏

Do you have seasonal allergies that require medical treatment? ❏ ❏

12. Do you use any special protective or corrective equipment or devices that aren't usually used for your sport or position (for example, knee brace, special neck roll, foot orthotics, retainer on your teeth, or hearing aid)? ❏ ❏

	YES	NO

13. Are you satisfied with your body shape and size? ❏ ❏

   What was your highest _____ and lowest _____
   body weight last year? ❏ ❏

   Have you ever been diagnosed with an eating disorder? ❏ ❏

14. Have you had problems with your eyes or vision? ❏ ❏

   Do you wear glasses, contacts, or protective eyewear? ❏ ❏

15. Do you have any other concerns you would like to discuss
   (e.g., social, academic, or family issues)? ❏ ❏

16. Many people feel depressed at times.

   Please rate any recent feelings of depression you may have had:

   Use a number from 0 (none) to 10 (severe) _____

17. Record the dates of your most recent immunization (shots) for:

   _____ Tetanus   _____ Measles/MMR

   _____ Hepatitis B   _____ Chicken pox

Females Only

18. When was your first menstrual period? _____

   When was your most recent menstrual period? _____

   How much time do you usually have from the
   start of one period to the start of another? _____

   How many periods have you had in the last year? _____

   Date of last pap/pelvic exam? _____

Explain "Yes" answers here:

_____

_____

_____

_____

_____

_____

I hereby state that, to the best of my knowledge, my answers to the above
questions are complete and correct.

Signature of athlete _____

Date _____

Weight History

Current Ht: _____ Current Wt: _____ (/ /)

If known:

Body fat % _____ (/ /) Method: _____

Usual Wt: _____ How long? _____

Personal goal wt: _____ Calculated IBW: _____

Highest wt: _____ When/How long: _____

Lowest wt: _____ When/How long: _____

Weight change with training/season?   Yes   No

Tried to control weight?   Yes   No

If yes, how? _____

_____

Training/Competition Schedule

When does your season start/end?

_____

_____

What is your weekly training schedule?

_____

_____

Do you participate in aerobic activities outside of your daily training schedule?

_____

_____

Weight Control History

Diet pills _____   Current   Past

Diuretics _____   Current   Past

Vomiting_____   Current   Past

Fasting _____   Current   Past

Laxatives_____   Current   Past

Exercise_____   Current   Past

Special Diet _____   Current   Past

Other: _____

_____

(continued)

Diet History

Meals/day: _____ Snacks/day: _____ Eating-out frequency: _____
Vit/min supplements: _____
Other supplements:_____

Food Frequency

	Daily	Weekly	Monthly
Red meat	_____	_____	_____
Poultry	_____	_____	_____
Fish	_____	_____	_____
Eggs	_____	_____	_____
Beans/lentils	_____	_____	_____
Milk	_____	_____	_____
Yogurt	_____	_____	_____
Cheese	_____	_____	_____
Vegetables	_____	_____	_____
Fruit	_____	_____	_____
Juice	_____	_____	_____
Soda	_____	_____	_____
Bread	_____	_____	_____
Cereal	_____	_____	_____
Rice	_____	_____	_____
Pasta	_____	_____	_____
Potatoes	_____	_____	_____
Fats	_____	_____	_____
Fried foods	_____	_____	_____
Peanut butter/nuts	_____	_____	_____
Candy	_____	_____	_____
Desserts	_____	_____	_____
Tea/coffee	_____	_____	_____
Alcohol	_____	_____	_____

How much water? _____
Avoid fat? _____
Forbidden foods?_____

UCLA Sports Medicine
Preparticipation Exam—Physical Exam

The following is the physical exam conducted by team physicians on all UCLA athletes.

Name _____ DOB _____

Sport _____ Vision R20/ _____ L20/ _____ Corrected: Y   N

Height _____ Weight _____

Pulse _____ BP _____/ _____ (_____/_____, _____/_____)

Medical	Normal	Abnormal	Initials
Appearance			
Eyes/Ears/Nose/Throat			
Lymph Nodes			
Heart			
Pulses			
Lungs			
Abdomen			
Genitalia (males only)			
Skin			
Muscoloskeletal	**Normal**	**Abnormal**	**Initials**
Neck			
Back			
Shoulder/Arm			
Elbow/Forearm			
Wrist/Hand			
Hip/Thigh			
Knee			
Leg/Ankle			
Foot			

(continued)

Assessment: ❏ Seat belts/Helmets
_____   ❏ Drinking/Driving
_____   ❏ ErOh/Tobacco
_____   ❏ Other drugs
Recommendations: ❏ Steroids/Supplements
_____   ❏ Safe sex
_____   ❏ Violence/Fights
_____   ❏ Weight control
Labs/Xrays:_____   ❏ Sun protection

Clearance Status

Cleared ❏   Date cleared: _____

Not cleared ❏   Reason: _____

❏ Immunizations given

_____

_____

                 Name of Physician (print/type)   Date

_____   _____

Signature of Physician_____

Permission was received to use the UCLA Sports Medicine Preparticipation Exam from the UCLA Division of Sports Medicine. This form is modified from the Preparticipation Physical Evaluation Monograph (Second Edition), published by the Physician and Sportsmedicine, 1997 and endorsed by the American Academy of Family Physicians, American Academy of Pediatrics, American Medical Society for Sports Medicine, American Osteopathic Academy of Sports Medicine.

appendix G

Sample Student-Athlete Contracts and Medical Release Authorizations

University of Utah Medical Information Release Authorization

This authorization is used by the University of Utah Student Athlete Wellness Team to prevent legal liability as well as promote an integrative eating disorder treatment approach and ensure open communication among all members of the eating disorder team.

University of Utah
Athletics Department

Authorization to Release Confidential/Medical Information

Effective Date: _____

Statement of Purpose

The University of Utah Athletics Department is devoted to the welfare of University of Utah student-athletes. The Athletics Department employs a full time Director of Student-Athlete Support Services to coordinate the services available to student-athletes and to assist and encourage student-athletes to utilize the services. The general healthcare services available include medical care, strength and fitness training, nutrition counseling and mental health counseling. The University of Utah personnel who provide such services work together as a Student Athlete Wellness Team with the goal of ensuring that student-athletes succeed in school and are fit to safely participate in intercollegiate athletics. To achieve this goal, it is critical that the Director of Student-Athlete Support Services have access to certain information concerning the physical and mental health of student-athletes.

Release

I, _____ authorize University of Utah team physicians, mental health counselors, trainers and other University of Utah affiliated medical personnel to discuss with each other and appropriate Athletics Department personnel, any injury, illness or condition that may affect my fitness to participate in intercollegiate athletics. I understand that I am eligible for all the same services offered at the University of Utah that are available to other University students.

_____

Signature

_____

Witness

_____

Date

University of California at Los Angeles
Student Athlete Contract

This student athlete contract is used by the UCLA Weight Management Team (medical staff) to ensure that the athlete follows appropriate treatment requirements. This particular contract is used specifically for athletes participating in cross-country and track; however, there are contracts available for all female athletic teams.

RE: CONTRACT FOR

FROM: The UCLA Medical Staff, Department of Intercollegiate Athletics

Dear

As you are aware, the members of the UCLA Sports Medicine Team have established some guidelines and recommendations to assist you with your health and well-being while participating as an athlete on the UCLA Women's Cross Country and Track Team. Based on our careful medical review of your health and desire to optimize your health and well-being, it is our opinion that you not train competitively for the remainder of this school year. It is our opinion that competitive training at this point in time may increase your risk for serious harm to your bone health and psychological well-being. In order to optimize your health and consider your return to a healthier state of training competitively, the following recommendations have been made, effective immediately:

1. Weekly appointments with Dr. _____ in the UCLA Student Psychological Services for individual therapy. At times, Dr. _____ may recommend biweekly therapy.

2. Weekly or biweekly appointments in the UCLA Outpatient Eating Disorder Program for group therapy. Presently, you are in the Phase I Program meeting one time per week. It is recommended that you enter the Phase II Program as soon as there is an opening at which time you will be meeting twice per week for 4 hours per session. It may be recommended that you enter an in-patient eating disorder program. This will be re-evaluated while you are in the Phase II Program by the eating disorder program staff and athletic team medical staff. Medications may be recommended by the medical staff to improve your well-being. A consult with Dr. _____ or other psychiatrist specializing in eating disorders may be needed periodically to assist with your medical therapy.

3. Weekly appointments with your nutritionist. Your goal is to keep in a state of a positive energy balance, eating a balanced diet of healthy foods, as recommended by your nutritionist and the medical staff you work with. Calcium intake recommendations include 1,500 mg per day of calcium with 400-800 IU per day of vitamin D.

(continued)

4. Every other week appointments with Dr. _____
   for a medical assessment and possible tests, including blood and urine
   tests if needed. Dr. _____ will be coordinating
   your care with the other members of the health care team. Medications
   may be recommended to help improve your bone health and to ensure
   monthly menstrual periods.

5. Maintenance of weight over 100 pounds. If weight falls below this
   level, weekly weight checks may be requested for optimal health and
   well-being.

6. Exercise activity, if desired, should not exceed 4 days per week, with the
   maximum recommended time of 30 minutes per session. High intensity
   activity is not recommended. Cross-training is recommended. Running,
   if desired, should not exceed 10 to 15 miles per week. It is recommended
   that on a daily basis you stay in a state of positive energy balance.

7. ATC will be assisting you and will be available to help coordinate your
   meetings with Dr. _____ and Dr. _____
   ___ if needed.

The above recommendations are the result of thoughtful discussions with
you and your health care team. We are committed to assisting you with your
health needs and look forward to working together with you. We will be
re-evaluating your medical health on a regular basis and at the end of the
school year. Changes may be made to the above recommendations prior to
the end of the school year. The recommendations have been made to assist
you with your present health care needs. Your participation on the UCLA
Women's Cross Country and Track Team for the _____ season
will be re-evaluated at the end of the school year. An assessment of your
medical health and well-being will be made at this time regarding whether
or not you will be able to safely participate on the team in the future. This
decision will be a collective recommendation by the UCLA eating disorder
medical staff and the UCLA sports medicine health care staff.

Sincerely,

Please sign below if you agree to follow the above guidelines and recommendations.

_____

Signature

_____

Date

Permission was received to use the UCLA Sports Medicine Preparticipation Exam from the UCLA Divi-
sion of Sports Medicine. This form is modified from the Preparticipation Physical Evaluation Monograph
(Second Edition), published by the Physician and Sportsmedicine, 1997 and endorsed by the American
Academy of Family Physicians, American Academy of Pediatrics, American Medical Society for Sports
Medicine, American Osteopathic Academy of Sports Medicine.

glossary

acid–base balance—A relative balance of acid and base products in the body so that optimal pH is maintained in the tissues, particularly the blood.

adrenal hormones—Hormones produced by the adrenal glands including the sex hormones (i.e., androgens and estrogens), glucocorticoid hormones (e.g., cortisol), and mineralocorticoid hormones (e.g., aldosterone).

aerobic—Relating to energy processes that occur in the presence of oxygen, generally during low-intensity exercise of long duration (i.e., endurance exercise).

aesthetic sports—Sports in which performance is judged, such as cheerleading, diving, figure skating, gymnastics, and synchronized swimming.

amenorrhea—Absence of menstruation.

anaerobic—Relating to energy processes that occur in the absence of oxygen, generally during high-intensity exercise of short duration.

anorexia athletica—A subclinical eating disorder identified in elite female athletes. The disorder is characterized by an intense fear of gaining weight or becoming fat even though underweight (at least 5% below the expected normal weight for age and height), severe energy restriction (<1,200 kcal/d), excessive exercise, self-induced vomiting, or the abuse of laxatives and diuretics.

anorexia nervosa—A clinical eating disorder characterized by extreme body image distortion and self-starvation.

anovulation—A form of menstrual dysfunction characterized by an absence of ovulation. The term may be used for abnormal cycle lengths ranging from very short cycles (< 21 days) to overly long cycles (35-150 days).

anthropometrics—Measurement of body mass and composition, as well as girth and diameter of body parts.

antidepressant—A drug used to prevent or treat depression.

basal metabolic rate (BMR)—The energy required to maintain bodily functions at rest.

body composition—The relative percentages of fat mass and fat-free mass.

body dysmorphic disorder—A body image disorder characterized by an intense and excessive preoccupation or dissatisfaction with a perceived defect in appearance.

body mass index (BMI)—A ratio of body weight (kg) relative to height (m^2) that is frequently used to assess obesity risk.

bulimia nervosa—A clinical eating disorder characterized by repeated cycles of bingeing and purging (at least twice a week for a period of at least three months).

cardiac output—A measurement of the blood flow through the heart to the systemic (and pulmonary) circulation. Cardiac output is expressed as volume of blood per unit of time or liters/minute.

catabolic—Relating to the breakdown of compounds and materials.

CONFRONT plan—A series of steps for approaching the individual with an eating disorder, developed by the National Association of Anorexia Nervosa and Associated Disorders.

cortisol—An adrenocortical hormone usually referred to pharmaceutically as hydrocortisone. Closely related to cortisone in physiological effects.

dehydration—A reduction of body water below normal levels, which generally occurs when water output exceeds water intake.

disordered eating—The spectrum of abnormal and harmful eating behaviors that are used in a misguided attempt to lose weight or maintain a lower-than-normal body weight.

eating disorder—One of three clinical eating disorders—anorexia nervosa, bulimia nervosa, and eating disorders not otherwise specified (EDNOS)—recognized in the American Psychiatric Association's (1994) *Diagnostic and Statistical Manual of Mental Disorders* (DSM-IV).

eating disorder not otherwise specified (EDNOS)—A clinical eating disorder category recently added to the DSM-IV (APA 1994) to describe a condition that meets some but not all of the criteria for anorexia nervosa and bulimia nervosa.

electrolyte—A substance that conducts an electrical current when in a solution; in the body, electrolytes function to regulate water balance.

endurance sports—Sports that involve prolonged aerobic activity, such as cross-country skiing, cycling, distance running, and swimming.

energy efficiency—A decrease in the energy required to perform a given task.

epinephrine—A hormone secreted by the adrenal medulla in response to splanchnic stimulation. Its effects are similar to those brought about by stimulation of the sympathetic division of the autonomic nervous system.

exercise therapy—A less well known form of adjunct treatment that focuses on using physical activity and movement to help treat a client with disordered eating.

experiential therapies—Alternative types of therapy that may involve some form of expressive art (e.g., dance, art, music) in the recovery process.

fat-free mass—The mass of the human body remaining after extraction of all fat; it generally includes bone, muscle tissue, body fluids, and vital organs.

fat mass—The lipid-containing portions of the body, including the essential fat (i.e., fat that is an essential part of tissues such as cell membranes, nerves sheaths, and the brain) and storage fat (i.e., fat that accumulates and is stored in the adipose tissues).

fight or flight response—A theory of the emotions, advanced by W.B. Cannon, that animal and human organisms respond to emergency situations by increased sympathetic nervous system activity, including an increased catecholamine production with associated increases in blood pressure, heart and respiratory rates, and skeletal muscle blood flow.

food efficiency—A decrease in the number of calories required to maintain a given body weight or composition.

hematuria—Blood in urine. Urine may be slightly smoky, reddish, or very red.

hemoglobin—The iron-containing pigment of the red blood cells. Its function is to carry oxygen from the lungs to the tissues. The amount of hemoglobin in the blood averages 12 to 16 g/100 ml in adult females, 14 to 18 g/100 ml in males, and somewhat less in children.

hemolysis—The destruction of red blood cells with the liberation of hemoglobin, which diffuses into the fluid surrounding them. When hemolysis occurs within the blood vessels, the body is unable to retain the hemoglobin, which is lost through the kidneys and imparts a red color to the urine.

hypokalemia—A decreased concentration of potassium in the blood.

hyponatremia—A decreased concentration of sodium in the blood.

immunoglobulin (ABBR Ig)—One of a family of closely related though not identical proteins that are capable of acting as antibodies. Five major types of immunoglobulins are normally present in the human adult: IgG, IgA, IgM, IgD, and IgE.

iron-deficiency anemia—The third stage of iron deficiency characterized by impaired hemoglobin synthesis and small, poorly developed red blood cells.

iron-deficiency erythropoiesis—The second stage of iron deficiency characterized by a decresed ability to synthesize new red blood cells.

leukocyte—White blood corpuscle. Leukocytes act as scavengers helping to combat infection.

luteal phase deficiency—A form of menstrual dysfunction characterized by a shortened luteal phase, which may or may not be accompanied by a prolonged follicular phase.

lymphocyte—Lymph cell or white blood corpuscle without cytoplasmic granules. They normally number from 20 to 50% of total white blood cells.

macronutrients—Carbohydrates, proteins, and fats.

melatonin—A hormone that is produced by the body in the greatest quantities at night, has been associated with a decrease in body temperature and feelings of sleepiness, and may be implicated in disordered eating behavior.

micronutrients—Vitamins and minerals.

monocyte—A large mononuclear leukocyte having more protoplasm than a lymphocyte.

muscle dysmorphia—A subtype of body dysmorphic disorder characterized by an inordinate preoccupation and dissatisfaction with body size and muscularity. Also known as the "Adonis complex."

myoglobin—A red iron-containing protein pigment in muscle tissue that serves as an oxygen carrier.

neutrophil—A leukocyte that stains easily with neutral dyes.

norepinephrine—A hormone produced by the adrenal medulla, similar in chemical properties and physiological effects to epinephrine.

nutritional rehabilitation—A part of treatment for disordered eating that focuses on educating a client about healthful eating patterns.

orthostatic hypotension—Postural hypotension: decrease in blood pressure upon assuming erect posture. This is normal, but may be of such degree as to cause fainting especially in persons that first stand up after having been flat in bed for several days.

osteopenia—A bone disorder characterized by a reduction in bone mineral density of between 1 and 2.5 standard deviations below the mean for age-matched individuals.

osteoporosis—A bone disorder characterized by a reduction in bone mineral density of more than 2.5 standard deviations below the mean for age-matched individuals. The bones become overly porous and highly susceptible to fracture.

overtraining syndrome—A condition seen in athletes who engage in excessive training, characterized by a marked decrease in performance and an increased risk for injury.

pharmacological treatment—A portion of treatment that may involve taking psychotropic medications (e.g., antidepressants) to treat underlying biological and genetic influences of a disorder.

preparticipation physical—Physical examination of athletes before their competitive season, which typically includes a general evaluation of body systems, completion of a health history, and sometimes assessment of urinary and blood chemistry.

primary amenorrhea—A form of menstrual dysfunction characterized by no menstrual period by the age of 16; also known as "delayed menarche."

psychosocial intervention—A type of treatment intervention that involves traditional psychotherapy (e.g., talk therapy) with a psychologist or counselor.

referral—A source for eating disorder treatment or information.

registered dietitian—A nutrition professional who has completed at least a four-year degree in nutrition from an accredited college, finished a clinical internship, and passed a comprehensive national registration exam.

secondary amenorrhea—A form of menstrual dysfunction characterized by the absence of three or more consecutive menstrual cycles.

self-report questionnaire—A form of assessment consisting of a compilation of questions that the respondent completes on his or her own.

serotonin—A neurotransmitter that plays a significant role in hunger and satiety and has been postulated to play a role in the development or maintenance of eating disorders, particularly bulimia nervosa.

serotonin hypothesis—The hypothesis that bulimia nervosa is the behavioral expression of decreased levels or activity of serotonin in the central nervous system (Goldbloom and Garfinkel 1990).

stroke volume—The amount of blood pumped by the heart with each heart beat, expressed in milliliters per beat.

structured interview—A form of assessment consisting of a series of questions that are delivered by an interviewer and answered by the respondent.

subclinical eating disorder—A disorder that involves considerable eating pathology and body weight concerns but no significant psychopathology or one that fails to meet all the DSM-IV (APA 1994) criteria for anorexia nervosa, bulimia nervosa, or EDNOS.

thin-build sports—Sports in which a low body weight is thought to confer a competitive advantage, either for aesthetic reasons or for speed and economy of movement, including aesthetic sports, endurance sports, and weight-dependent sports.

$\dot{V}O_2$**max**—Maximal oxygen uptake, measured during exercise. It reflects the body's ability to utilize oxygen at the cellular level and is an indication of aerobic fitness.

weight-cutting—A practice common among wrestlers in which large amounts of weight are lost (via unhealthy or pathogenic means) in a short period of time so that the wrestler can compete in a lower weight class.

weight cycling—Repeated cycles of losing and regaining weight.

weight-dependent sports—Sports that use weight classifications, such as bodybuilding, jockeying, karate, light-weight rowing, powerlifting, and wrestling.

references

American College of Sports Medicine. 1996. Position stand: Weight loss in wrestlers. *Medicine and Science in Sports and Exercise* 28:ix-xii.

American Psychiatric Association (APA). 1994. *Diagnostic and statistical manual of mental disorders.* 4th ed. Washington, DC: American Psychiatric Association.

———. 1999. *Developing a treatment plan for the individual patient.* [Online]. Available: www.psych.org/clin_res/guide.bk-3.cfm.

———. 2000. Practice guideline for the treatment of patients with eating disorders. *American Journal of Psychiatry* 157 (1 Suppl.): 1-39.

Andersen, A.E. 1992. Eating disorders in male athletes: A special case? In *Eating, body weight and performance in athletes: Disorders of modern society,* ed. K.D. Brownell, J. Rodin, and J.H. Wilmore, 172-188. Philadelphia: Lea and Febiger.

———. 2001. Progress in eating disorders research. *American Journal of Psychiatry* 158:515-517.

Andersen, A., T. Gray, and J. Holman. 1996. Osteopenia in males with eating disorders. In *Seventh International Conference on Eating Disorders.* New York.

Andersen, A.E., and J.E. Holman. 1997. Males with eating disorders: Challenges for treatment and research. *Psychopharmacology Bulletin* 33:391-397.

Andersen, A.E., T. Watson, and J. Schlechte. 2000. Osteoporosis and osteopenia in men with eating disorders. *Lancet* 355:1967-1968.

Andersen, A.E., P.J. Woodward, and N. LaFrance. 1995. Bone mineral density of eating disorder subgroups. *International Journal of Eating Disorders* 18:335-342.

Andersen, G.H. 1996. Hunger, appetite, and food intake. In *Present Knowledge in Nutrition, 7th edition,* ed. E.E. Ziegler and L.J. Filer. Washington, DC: ILSI Press.

Apfelbaum, M., J. Bostsarron, and D. Lucatis. 1971. Effect of caloric restriction and excessive caloric intake on energy expenditure. *American Journal of Clinical Nutrition* 24:1405-1409.

Arena, B., N. Maffulli, F. Maffulli, and M.A. Morleo. 1995. Reproductive hormones and menstrual changes with exercise in female athletes. *Sports Medicine* 19:278-287.

Astrup, A., P.C. Gotzsche, K. van de Werken, C. Ranneries, S. Toubro, A. Raben, and B. Buemann. 1999. Meta-analysis of resting metabolic rate in formerly obese subjects. *American Journal of Clinical Nutrition* 69:1117-1122.

Baumann, J. 1992. Reflections on group psychotherapy with eating-disordered patients. *Group* 16 (2): 95-100.

Beals, K. 2002. Body dissatisfaction and disordered eating among triathletes. Southwest American College of Sports Medicine, annual meeting, November 2002. Abstract.

Beals, K.A., and M.M. Manore. 1994. The prevalence and consequences of subclinical eating disorders in female athletes. *International Journal of Sport Nutrition* 4:175-195.

———. 1998. Nutritional status of female athletes with subclinical eating disorders. *Journal of the American Dietetic Association* 98:419-425.

———. 1999. Subclinical eating disorders in active women. *Topics in Clinical Nutrition* 14:14-24.

———. 2000. Behavioral, psychological and physical characteristics of female athletes with subclinical eating disorders. *International Journal of Sport Nutrition and Exercise Metabolism* 10:128-143.

———. 2002. Disorders of the female athlete triad among collegiate athletes. *International Journal of Sport Nutrition and Exercise Metabolism* 12:281-293.

Beckvid-Henriksson, G., C. Schnell, and A. Linden-Hirschberg. 2000. Women endurance runners with menstrual dysfunction have prolonged interruption of training due to injury. *Gynecologic and Obstetric Investigation* 49:41-46.

Beumont, P.J.V., B. Arthur, J.D. Russell, and S.W. Touyz. 1994. Excessive physical activity in dieting disorder patients: Proposals for a supervised exercise program. *International Journal of Eating Disorders* 15 (1): 21-36.

Black, D.R., and M.E. Burkes-Miller. 1988. Male and female college athletes: Use of anorexia nervosa and bulimia nervosa weight loss methods. *Research Quarterly* 59: 252-259.

Black, D.R., L.J.S. Larkin, D.C. Coster, L.J. Leverenz, and D.A. Abood. In press. Physiologic screening test for eating disorders/disordered eating for female collegiate athletes. *Journal of Athletic Training*.

Blinder, B.J., D.M. Freeman, and A.J. Stunkard. 1970. Behavior therapy of anorexia nervosa: Effectiveness of activity as a reinforcer of weight gain. *American Journal of Psychiatry* 126 (8): 1093-1098.

Blouin, A.G., and G.S. Goldfield. 1995. Body image and steroid use in male bodybuilders. *International Journal of Eating Disorders* 18:159-165.

Boachie, A., G.S. Goldfield, and W. Spettigue. 2003. Olanzapine use as an adjunctive treatment: Hospitalized children with anorexia nervosa: Case reports. *International Journal of Eating Disorders* 33 (1): 98-103.

Bo-Linn, G.W. 1986. Understanding medical complications in eating disorders. In *Eating disorders*, ed. F.E.F. Larocca, 5-12. San Francisco: Jossey-Bass.

Bonen, A., A. Belcastro, W.Y. Ling, and A.A. Simpson. 1981. Profiles of selected hormones during menstrual cycles of teenage athletes. *Journal of Applied Physiology* 50:545-551.

Boskind-White, M., and W.C. White. 1987. *Bulimarexia: The binge/purge cycle.* 2nd ed. New York: Norton.

Bowers, T.K., and E. Eckert. 1978. Leukopenia in anorexia nervosa: Lack of increased risk of infection. *Archives of Internal Medicine* 138:1520-1526.

Boyle, P.C., L.H. Storlien, and R.E. Keesey. 1978. Increased efficiency of food utilization following weight loss. *Physiology and Behavior* 21:261-264.

Brook, C.G.D., and N.J. Marshal. 1996. *Essential endocrinology.* 3rd ed. Oxford: Blackwell Science.

Brooks-Gunn, J., M.P. Warren, and L.H. Hamilton. 1987. The relation of eating problems and amenorrhea in ballet dancers. *Medicine and Science in Sports and Exercise* 19:41-44.

Brownell, K.D., and J.P. Foryet, eds. 1986. *Handbook of eating disorders: Physiology, psychology, and treatment of obesity, anorexia nervosa, and bulimia nervosa.* New York: Basic Books.

Brownell, K.D., and J. Rodin. 1992. Prevalence of eating disorders in athletes. In *Eating, body weight and performance in athletes: Disorders of modern society*, ed. K.D. Brownell, J. Rodin, and J.H. Wilmore, 128-145. Philadelphia: Lea and Febiger.

Brownell, K.D., S.N. Steen, and J.H. Wilmore. 1987. Weight regulation practices in athletes: Analysis of metabolic and health effects. *Medicine and Science in Sports and Exercise* 19:546-556.

Brumberg, J.J. 1988. *Fasting girls: The history of anorexia nervosa.* New York: Plume.

Bruno, A., N. Maffulli, F. Maffulli, and M.A. Morleo. 1995. Reproductive hormones and menstrual changes with exercise in female athletes. *Sports Medicine* 19:278-287.

Bunnell, D.W., I.R. Shenker, M.P. Nussbaum, M.S. Jacobson, and P. Cooper. 1990. Subclinical versus formal eating disorders: Differentiating psychological features. *International Journal of Eating Disorders* 9 (3): 357-362.

Button, E.J., and A. Whitehouse. 1981. Subclinical anorexia nervosa. *Psychological Medicine* 11:509-516.

Byrne, S., and N. McLean. 2001. Eating disorders in athletes: A review of the literature. *Journal of Science and Medicine in Sport* 4:145-159.

Carek, P.J., and M. Futrell. 1999. Athlete's view of the preparticipation physical exam. *Archives of Family Medicine* 8:307-312.

Carney, C.P., and A.E. Andersen. 1996. Eating disorders: Guide to medical evaluation and complications. *Psychiatric Clinics of North America* 19:657-679.

Carson, J.D., and E. Bridges. 2001. Abandoning routine body composition assessment: A strategy to reduce disordered eating among female athletes and dancers. Canadian Academy of Sport Medicine position statement. *Clinical Journal of Sports Medicine* 11:280.

Carter, J.C., D.A. Stewart, and C.G. Fairburn. 1998. The primary prevention of eating disorders: The dilemma and its denial. *Eating Disorders: The Journal of Treatment and Prevention* 6:213-215.

Castro, J., L. Lazaro, F. Pons, I. Halperin, and J. Toro. 2000. Predictors of bone mineral density reduction in adolescents with anorexia nervosa. *Journal of the American Academy of Child and Adolescent Psychiatry* 39:1365-1370.

Castro, J., J. Toro, L. Lazaro, F. Pons, and I. Halperin. 2002. Bone mineral density in male adolescents with anorexia nervosa. *Journal of the American Academy of Child and Adolescent Psychiatry* 41:613-618.

Chapman, P., R.B. Toma, R.V. Tuveson, and M. Jacob. 1997. Nutrition knowledge among adolescent high school female athletes. *Adolescence* 32:437-446.

Clark, D., F. Thomas, R.T. Withers, M. Brinkman, C. Chandler, J. Phillips, J. Ballard, M.N. Berry, and P. Nestel. 1992. Differences in energy metabolism between normal weight "large eating" and "small eating" women. *British Journal of Nutrition* 68:31-44.

Clark, N., M. Nelson, and W. Evans. 1988. Nutrition education for elite female runners. *Physician and Sportsmedicine* 16 (2): 124-136.

Constantini, N.A. 1994. Clinical consequences of athletic amenorrhea. *Sports Medicine* 17:213-223.

Convertino, V.A., L.E. Armstrong, E.F. Coyle, G.W. Mack, M.N. Swaka, L.C. Senay, and W.M. Sherman. 1996. ACSM position stand: Exercise and fluid replacement. *Medicine and Science in Sports and Exercise* 28:i-vii.

Coogan, A.R., and E.F. Coyle. 1987. Reversal of fatigue during prolonged exercise by carbohydrate infusion or ingestion. *Journal of Applied Physiology* 63:2388-2395.

Cooper, P.J., M.J. Taylor, Z. Cooper, and C.G. Fairburn. 1987. The development and validation of the body shape questionnaire. *International Journal of Eating Disorders* 6 (4):485-494.

Cooper, Z., and C.G. Fairburn. 1987. The eating disorder examination: A semi-structured interview for the assessment of the specific psychopathology of eating disorders. *International Journal of Eating Disorders* 6:1-8.

Corley, G., M. Menarest-Litchford, and T.L. Bazzarre. 1990. Nutrition knowledge and dietary practices of college coaches. *Journal of the American Dietetic Association* 90: 705-709.

Costill, D.L. 1988. Carbohydrate for exercise: Dietary demands for optimal performance. *International Journal of Sports Medicine* 9:1-18.

Costin, C. 1999. *The eating disorder sourcebook*. 2nd ed. Lincolnwood, IL: Lowell House.

Coyle, E.F. 1995. Substrate utilization during exercise in active people. *American Journal of Clinical Nutrition* 61 (Suppl.): 968S-979S.

Craig, A.R., J.A. Franklin, and G. Andrews. 1984. A scale to measure locus of control behavior. *British Journal of Medical Psychology* 57:173-180.

Crisp, A.H. 1967. Anorexia nervosa. *Hospital Medicine* 1:713-718.

————. 1983. Some aspects of the psychopathology of anorexia nervosa. In *Anorexia nervosa: Recent developments in research*, ed. P.L. Darby, P.E. Garfinkel, D.M. Garner, D.C. Coscina, 15-28. New York: Alan Liss.

Crisp, A.H., and D.A. Toms. 1972. Primary anorexia nervosa or weight phobia in the male: A report on 13 cases. *British Medical Journal* 1:334-338.

Curran-Celentano, J., J.W. Erdman, R.A. Nelson, and S.J.E. Grater. 1985. Alterations in vitamin A and thyroid hormone status in anorexia nervosa and associated disorders. *American Journal of Clinical Nutrition* 42:1183-1189.

Dale, K.S., and D.M. Landers. 1999. Weight control in wrestlers: Eating disorders or disordered eating? *Medicine and Science in Sports and Exercise* 31:1382-1389.

Dally, P. 1969. *Anorexia nervosa*. London: Heinemann Medical Books.

Davis, C. 1990. Body image and weight preoccupation: A comparison between exercising and non-exercising women. *Appetite* 15:13-21.

Davis, C., and M. Cowles. 1989. A comparison of weight and diet concerns and personality factors among female athletes and non-athletes. *Journal of Psychosomatic Research* 33:527-536.

De Caprio, C., F. Pasanisi, and F. Contaldo. 2000. Gastrointestinal complications in a patient with eating disorders. *Eating and Weight Disorders* 5:228-230.

Dick, R.W. 1991. Eating disorders in NCAA athletic programs. *Athletic Training* 26: 137-140.

Drenowski, A., and D.K. Yee. 1987. Men and body image. Are males satisfied with their body weight? *Psychosomatic Medicine* 49:626-634.

Drinkwater, B.L. 1992. Amenorrhea, body weight, and osteoporosis. In *Eating, body weight and performance in athletes: Disorders of modern society*, ed. K.D. Brownell, J. Rodin, and J.H. Wilmore, 235-247. Philadelphia: Lea and Febiger.

Drinkwater, B.L., B. Bruemmer, and C.H. Chestnut. 1990. Menstrual history as a determinant of current bone density in young athletes. *Journal of the American Medical Association* 263:545-548.

Drinkwater, B.L., K. Nilson, C.H. Chestnut, W.J. Bremner, S. Shainholtz, and M.B. Southworth. 1984. Bone mineral content of amenorrheic and eumenorrheic athletes. *New England Journal of Medicine* 31:277-281.

Drinkwater, B.L., K. Nilson, S. Ott, and C.H. Chestnut. 1986. Bone mineral density after resumption of menses in amenorrheic athletes. *Journal of the American Medical Association* 18:380-382.

Dueck, C.A., M.M. Manore, and K.S. Matt. 1996. Role of energy balance in athletic menstrual dysfunction. *International Journal of Sport Nutrition* 6:90-116.

Dummer, G.M., J.W. Rosen, W.W. Hensner, P.J. Roberts, and J.E. Counsilman. 1987. Pathogenic weight control behaviors of young competitive swimmers. *Physician and Sportsmedicine* 15 (5): 75-84.

Eichner, E.R. 1992. General health issues of low body weight and undereating in athletes.

In *Eating, body weight and performance in athletes: Disorders of modern society,* ed. K.D. Brownell, J. Rodin, and J.H. Wilmore, 191-201. Philadelphia: Lea and Febiger.

Epling, W.F., and W.D. Pierce. 1988. Activity-based anorexia nervosa. *International Journal of Eating Disorders* 7:475-485.

Epling, W.F., W.D. Pierce, and L. Stefan. 1993. A theory of activity-based anorexia nervosa. *International Journal of Eating Disorders* 3:27-46.

Evers, C.L. 1989. Dietary intake and symptoms of anorexia nervosa in female university dancers. *Journal of the American Dietetic Association* 89:98-100.

Fairburn, C.G., and K.D. Brownell, eds. 2001. *Eating disorders and obesity: A comprehensive handbook.* 2nd ed. New York: Guilford Press.

Fairburn, C.G., and Z. Cooper. 1993. The eating disorder examination. In *Binge eating: Nature, assessment, and treatment,* 12th ed., 3-14. New York: Guilford Press.

Fairburn, C.G., S.L. Welch, H.A. Doll, B.A. Davies, and M.E. O'Connor. 1997. Risk factors for bulimia nervosa: A community-based, case-control study. *Archives of General Psychiatry* 54:509-517.

Field, A.E., L. Cheung, A.M. Wolf, D.B. Herzog, S.L. Gortmaker, and G.A. Colditz. 1999. Exposure to the mass media and weight concerns among adolescent girls. *Pediatrics* 103:1-5.

Fogelholm, M. 1994. Effects of body weight reduction on sports performance. *Sports Medicine* 4:259-267.

Fogelholm, M., and H. Hilloskorpi. 1999. Weight and diet concerns in Finnish female and male athletes. *Medicine and Science in Sports and Exercise* 31:229-235.

Fries, H. 1974. Secondary amenorrhea, self-induced weight reduction, and anorexia nervosa. *Acta Psychiatrica Scandinavica* (Suppl.) 248:1-70.

Gadpille, W.J., C.F. Sanborn, and W.W. Wagner. 1987. Athletic amenorrhea, major affective disorders and eating disorders. *American Journal of Psychiatry* 144:939-942.

Garfinkel, P.E. 1996. Multimodal therapies for anorexia nervosa. In *Treating eating disorders,* ed. J. Werne. San Francisco: Jossey-Bass.

Garfinkel, P.E., D.M. Garner, and D.S. Goldbloom. 1987. Eating disorders: Implications for the 1990's. *Canadian Journal of Psychiatry* 32: 624-631.

Garner, D.M. 1991. *Eating Disorder Inventory-2 manual.* Odessa, FL: Psychological Assessment Resources.

Garner, D.M., and P.E. Garfinkel. 1979. The Eating Attitudes Test: An index of the symptoms of anorexia nervosa. *Psychological Medicine* 9:273-279.

———. 1980. Sociocultural factors in the development of anorexia nervosa. *Psychological Medicine* 10:647-656.

Garner, D.M., M.P. Olmstead, Y. Bohr, and P.E. Garfinkel. 1982. The Eating Attitudes Test: Psychometric features and clinical correlates. *Psychological Medicine* 12:871-878.

Garner, D.M., M.P. Olmstead, and J. Polivy. 1983. Development and validation of a multidimensional eating disorder inventory for anorexia nervosa and bulimia. *International Journal of Eating Disorders* 2 (2): 15-34.

Garner, D.M., and L.W. Rosen. 1991. Eating disorders among athletes: Research and recommendations. *Journal of Applied Sport Science Research* 5:100-107.

Garner, D.M., L.W. Rosen, and D. Barry. 1998. Eating disorders among athletes: Research and recommendations. *Sport Psychiatry* 7:839-857.

Gleaves, D.H., K.J. Miller, T.L. Williams, and S.A. Summers. 2000. Eating disorders: An overview. In *Comparative treatments for eating disorders,* ed. K.J. Miller and J.S. Mizes. New York: Springer.

Gold, P.W., H. Gwirtsman, P.C. Avgerinos, L.K. Nieman, W.T. Gallucci, W. Kaye, D. Jimerson, M. Ebert, R. Rittmaster, and D.L. Loriaux. 1986. Abnormal hypothalamic-pituitary-adrenal function in anorexia nervosa. *New England Journal of Medicine* 314: 1334-1342.

Goldberg, D.P., B. Cooper, M.R. Eastwood, H.B. Kedward, and M. Shepherd. 1970. A standardized psychiatric interview for use in community surveys. *British Journal of Preventive and Social Medicine* 24:18-23.

Goldbloom, D.S., and P.E. Garfinkel. 1990. The serotonin hypothesis of bulimia nervosa: Theory and evidence. *Canadian Journal of Psychiatry* 35:741-744.

Goldner, E. 1989. Treatment refusal in anorexia nervosa. *International Journal of Eating Disorders* 8 (3): 297-306.

Goldner, E.M., C.L. Birmingham, and V. Smye. 1997. Addressing treatment refusal in anorexia nervosa: Clinical, ethical, and legal considerations. In *Handbook of treatment for eating disorders*, ed. D.M. Garner and P.E. Garfinkel. New York: Guilford Press.

Goodsitt, A. 1997. Eating disorders: A self-psychological perspective. In *Handbook of treatment for eating disorders*, ed. D.M. Garner and P.E. Garfinkel. New York: Guilford.

Gottlieb, A.A., P.D. Smith, E.R. Cleveland, E.L. Flick, and J.P. Capps. 1994. Eating disorders and alcohol use among adolescent female cheerleaders [abstract]. *Journal of Adolescent Health* 15:80.

Greenleaf, J.E. 1992. Problem: Thirst, drinking behavior, and involuntary dehydration. *Medicine and Science in Sports and Exercise* 24:645-656.

Griffith, R.D., R.H. Dressendorfer, C.D. Fullbright, and C.E. Wade. 1990. Testicular function during exhaustive endurance training. *Physician and Sportsmedicine* 18:54-62.

Guthrie, S.R. 1991. Prevalence of eating disorders among intercollegiate athletes: Contributing factors and preventive measures. In *Eating disorders among athletes: Theory, issues, and research*, ed. D.R. Black, 43-66. Reston, VA: Association for the Advancement of Health Education and National Association for Girls and Women in Sport, Associations of the American Alliance for Health, Physical Education, Recreation, and Dance.

Hall, L., and M. Ostroff. 1999. *Anorexia nervosa: A guide to recovery*. Carlsbad, CA: Gurze.

Hamilton, L.H., J. Brooks-Gunn, and M.P. Warren. 1985. Sociocultural influences on eating disorders in professional female ballet dancers. *International Journal of Eating Disorders* 4:465-477.

Hamilton, L.H., J. Brooks-Gunn, M.P. Warren, and W.G. Hamilton. 1988. The role of selectivity in the pathogenesis of eating problems in ballet dancers. *Medicine and Science in Sports and Exercise* 20:560-565.

Harrison, K., and J. Cantor. 1997. The relationship between media consumption and eating disorders. *Journal of Communication* 47:40-67.

Herzog, D.B., I.S. Bradburn, and K. Newman. 1990. Sexuality in males with eating disorders. In *Males with eating disorders*, ed. A. Andersen, 40-53. New York: Brunner/Mazel.

Herzog, D.B., D.K. Norman, C. Gordon, and M. Pepose. 1984. Sexual conflict and eating disorders in 27 males. *American Journal of Psychiatry* 141:989-990.

Hill, L. 2001. *The Ohio State University Department of Athletics eating disorder policy 2001*. [Online]. Available: http://ohiostatebuckeyes.ocsn.com/genrel/sa-handbook/conduct.PDF.

Hinton, P.S., C. Giordano, T. Brownlie, and J.D. Haas. 2000. Iron supplementation improves endurance after training in iron-depleted, non-anemic women. *Journal of Applied Physiology* 88:1103-1111.

Hobbs, M., S. Birtchnell, A. Harte, and H. Lacey. 1989. Therapeutic factors in short-term group therapy for women with bulimia. *International Journal of Eating Disorders* 8 (6): 623-633.

Hoek, H.W. 1993. Review of the epidemiological studies on eating disorders. *International Review of Psychiatry* 5:61-74.

———. 1995. The distribution of eating disorders. In *Eating disorders and obesity: A comprehensive handbook,* ed. K.D. Brownell and C.G. Fairburn, 207-211. New York: Guilford Press.

Holliman, S.C. 1991. *Eating disorders and athletes: A handbook for coaches.* Dubuque, IA: American Alliance for Health, Physical Education, Recreation and Dance.

Hornyak, L.M., and E.K. Baker. 1989. Introduction. In *Experiential therapies for eating disorders,* ed. L.M. Hornyak and E.K. Baker. New York: Guilford.

Houtkooper, L. 2000. Body composition. In *Sport nutrition for health and performance,* ed. M.M. Manore and J.L. Thompson, 197-216. Champaign, IL: Human Kinetics.

Hsu, L.K.G. 1990. *Eating disorders.* New York: Guilford Press.

Hudson, J.I., H.G. Pope, and W.P. Carter. 1999. Pharmacologic therapy of bulimia nervosa. In *The management of eating disorders and obesity,* ed. D.J. Goldstein. Totawa, NJ: Humana.

Hulley, A.J., and A.J. Hill. 2001. Eating disorders and health in elite women distance runners. *International Journal of Eating Disorders* 30:312-317.

Ingjer, F., and J. Sundgot-Borgen. 1991. Influence of body weight reduction on maximal oxygen uptake in female elite athletes. *Scandinavian Journal of Medicine and Science in Sport* 1:141-146.

Jacobson, B.H., C. Sobonya, and J. Ransone. 2001. Nutrition practices and knowledge of college varsity athletes: A follow-up. *Journal of Strength and Conditioning Research* 15:63-68.

Johnson, C., P.S. Powers, and R. Dick. 1999. Athletes and eating disorders: The National Collegiate Athletic Association study. *International Journal of Eating Disorders* 26: 179-188.

Johnson, M.D. 1992. Tailoring the preparticipation exam to the female athletes. *Physician and Sportsmedicine* 20 (7): 61-72.

———. 1994. Disordered eating in active and athletic women. *Clinics in Sports Medicine* 13:355-369.

Joy, E., N. Clark, M.L. Ireland, J. Martire, A. Nattiv, and S. Varechok. 1997a. Team management of the female athlete triad. Roundtable. Part 1. What to look for? What to ask? *Physician and Sportsmedicine* 25:55-69.

———. 1997b. Team management of the female athlete triad. Roundtable. Part 2. Optimal treatment and prevention tactics. *Physician and Sportsmedicine* 25:94-110.

Kahm, A. 2001. Recovery through nutritional counseling. In *Eating disorders: New directions in treatment and recovery,* 2nd ed., ed. B.P. Kinovy. New York: Columbia.

Kaplan, H.I., and B.J. Sadock. 1998. *Synopsis of psychiatry.* 8th ed. Baltimore: Williams and Wilkins.

Kaye, W.H. 1999. Pharmacologic therapy for anorexia nervosa. In *The management of eating disorders and obesity,* ed. D.J. Goldstein. Totawa, NJ: Humana.

Kaye, W.H., and T.E. Weltzin. 1991. Serotonin activity in anorexia and bulimia nervosa: Relationship to the modulation of feeding and mood. *Journal of Clinical Psychiatry* 52 (Suppl.): 41-48.

Kellner, R., and B.F. Sheffield. 1973. A self-rating scale of distress. *Psychological Medicine* 3: 88-100.

Kennedy, S.H. 1994. Melatonin disturbances in anorexia nervosa and bulimia nervosa. *International Journal of Eating Disorders* 16 (3): 257-265.

Keys, A., J. Brozek, A. Henschel, O. Mickelsen, and H.L. Taylor. 1950. *The biology of human starvation.* Vol. 2. Minneapolis: University of Minnesota Press.

Killen, J.D., C.B. Taylor, L.D. Hammer, I. Litt, D.M. Wilson, T. Rich, C. Hayward, B. Simmonds, H. Kraemer, and A. Varady. 1993. An attempt to modify unhealthful eating attitudes and weight regulation practices of young adolescent girls. *International Journal of Eating Disorders* 13:369-384.

King, M.B., and G. Mezey. 1987. Eating behaviour of male race jockeys. *Psychological Medicine* 17:249-253.

Kurtzman, F.D., J. Yager, J. Landsverk, E. Wiesmeier, and D.C. Bodurka. 1989. Eating disorders among selected female student populations at UCLA. *Journal of the American Dietetic Association* 89:45-53.

Lackstrom, J.B., and D.B. Woodside. 1998. Families, therapists and family therapy in eating disorders. In *Treating eating disorders: Ethical, legal and personal issues,* ed. W. Vandereycken and P.J.V. Beumont. New York: New York University.

Lacy, C.F., L.L. Armstrong, M.P. Goldman, and L.L. Lance. 2002. *Drug information handbook.* Hudson, OH: Lexi-Comp.

Lankin, J.A., S.N. Steen, and R.A. Oppliger. 1990. Eating behaviors, weight loss methods, and nutrition practices among high school wrestlers. *Journal of Community Health Nursing* 7:223-234.

Laube, J.J. 1990. Why group therapy for bulimia? *International Journal of Group Psychotherapy* 40 (2): 169-187.

Le Grange, D., J. Tibbs, and T.D. Noakes. 1994. Implications of a diagnosis of anorexia nervosa in a ballet school. *International Journal of Eating Disorders* 15:369-376.

Leibel, R.L., M. Rosenbaum, and J. Hirsch. 1995. Changes in energy expenditure resulting from altered body weight. *New England Journal of Medicine* 332:621-628.

Lemon, P. 1995. Do athletes need more dietary protein and amino acids? *International Journal of Sport Nutrition* 5:S39-S61.

Leydon, M.A., C. Wall. 2002. New Zealand jockeys' dietary habits and their potential impact on health. *International Journal of Sport Nutrition and Exercise Metabolism* 12: 220-237.

Loucks, A.B., M. Verdun, and E.M. Heath. 1998. Low energy availability, not stress of exercise, alters LH pulsality of exercising women. *Journal of Applied Physiology* 84: 37-46.

Lukaski, H., C.B. Hall, and W.A. Siders. 1991. Altered metabolic response of iron deficient women during graded maximal exercises. *European Journal of Applied Sports Medicine* 63:140-145.

Lundholm, J.K., and J.M. Littrell. 1986. Desire for thinness among high school cheerleaders: Relationship to disordered eating and weight control behaviors. *Adolescence* 21:573-579.

Mann, T., S. Nolen-Hoeksema, K. Huang, D. Burgard, A. Wright, and K. Hanson. 1997. Are two interventions worse than none? Joint primary and secondary prevention of eating disorders in college females. *Health Psychology* 16:297-305.

Manore, M.M. 1996. Chronic dieting in active women: What are the health consequences? *Women's Health Issues* 6:332-341.

———. 1998. Running on empty: Chronic dieting in active women. *ACSM's Health and Fitness Journal* 2:24-31.

Manore, M.M., and J.L. Thompson. 2000. *Sport nutrition for health and performance.* Champaign, IL: Human Kinetics.

Marcus, R., C.E. Cann, P. Madvig, J. Minkoff, and M. Goodard. 1985. Menstrual function and bone mass in elite women distance runners. *Annals of Internal Medicine* 102:158-163.

Marshall, J.D., and V.J. Harber. 1996. Body dissatisfaction and drive for thinness in high performance field hockey athletes. *International Journal of Sports Medicine* 17: 541-544.

Martin, J.E. 1998. *Eating disorders, food, and occupational therapy.* London: Whurr.

Maughan, R.J. 1992. Fluid balance and exercise. *International Journal of Sports Medicine* 13:S132-S135.

McLean, J.A., S.I. Barr, and J.C. Prior. 2001. Dietary restraint, exercise, and bone density in young women: Are they related? *Medicine and Science in Sports and Exercise* 33: 1292-1296.

McNulty, K.Y., C.H. Adams, J.M. Anderson, and S.G. Affenito. 2001. Development and validation of a screening tool to identify eating disorders in female athletes. *Journal of the American Dietetic Association* 101:886-892.

Mickalide, A.D. 1990. Sociocultural factors influencing weight among males. In *Males with eating disorders,* ed. A. Andersen, 30-39. New York: Brunner/Mazel.

Morenoff, A., and B. Sobol. 1989. Art therapy in the long-term psychodynamic treatment of bulimic women. In *Experiential therapies for eating disorders,* ed. L.M. Hornyak and E.K. Baker. New York: Guilford.

Mulligan, K., and G.E. Butterfield. 1990. Discrepancies between energy intake and expenditure in physically active women. *British Journal of Nutrition* 64:23-36.

Munoz, M.T., and J. Argente. 2002. Anorexia nervosa in female adolescents: Endocrine and bone mineral density disturbances. *European Journal of Endocrinology* 147:275-286.

Muscari, M. 2002. Effective management of adolescents with anorexia and bulimia. *Journal of Psychosocial Nursing* 40 (2): 23-31.

Myburgh, K.H., J. Hutchins, A.B. Fataar, S.F. Hough, and T.D. Noakes. 1990. Low bone density is an etiologic factor for stress fractures in athletes. *Annals of Internal Medicine* 113:754-759.

Nagel, D.L., D.R. Black, L.J. Leverenz, and D.C. Coster. 2000. Evaluation of a screening test for female college athletes with eating disorders and disordered eating. *Journal of Athletic Training* 35:431-440.

Nattiv, A., R. Agostini, B. Drinkwater, and K.K. Yeager. 1994. The female athlete triad: The inter-relatedness of disordered eating, amenorrhea, and osteoporosis. *Clinics in Sports Medicine* 13:405-418.

Nattiv, A., and L. Lynch. 1994. The female athlete triad: Managing an acute risk to long-term health. *Physician and Sportsmedicine* 22 (1): 60-68.

Newhouse, I.J., and D.B. Clement. 1995. The efficacy of iron supplementation in iron depleted women. In *Sports nutrition: Vitamins and trace elements,* ed. I. Wolinsky and J. Driskell, 47-57. Boca Raton, FL: CRC Press.

Nichols, M.P., and R.C. Schwartz. 1995. *Family therapy: Concepts and methods.* 3rd ed. Needham Heights, MA: Allyn and Bacon.

Nielson, P., and D. Nachtigall. 1998. Iron supplementation in athletes: Current recommendations. *Sports Medicine* 26:207-216.

Noakes, T. 2002. Hyponatremia in distance runners: fluid and sodium balance during exercise. *Current Sports Medicine Reports* 1:197-207.

O'Connor, P.J., R.D. Lewis, and E.M. Kirchner. 1995. Eating disorder symptoms in female college gymnasts. *Medicine and Science in Sports and Exercise* 27:550-555.

O'Connor, P.J., and J.C. Smith. 1999. Physical activity and eating disorders. In *Lifestyle medicine*, ed. J.M. Rippe, 1005-1015. Oxford: Blackwell Science.

O'Keefe, K.A., R.E. Keith, G.D. Wilson, and D.L. Blessing. 1989. Dietary carbohydrate intake and endurance exercise in trained female cyclists. *Nutrition Research* 5:25-36.

Olivardia, R., H.G. Pope, and J.I. Hudson. 2000. Muscle dysmorphia in male weightlifters: A case–control study. *American Journal of Psychiatry* 157:1291-1296.

Olson, M.S., H.N. Williford, L.A. Richards, J.A. Brown, and S. Pugh. 1996. Self-reports on the Eating Disorder Inventory by female aerobic instructors. *Perceptual and Motor Skills* 82:1051-1058.

Oppliger, R.A., G.L. Landry, S.W. Foster, and A.C. Lambrecht. 1993. Bulimic behaviors among interscholastic wrestlers: A statewide survey. *Pediatrics* 91:826-831.

Otis, C.L. 1992. Exercise-associated amenorrhea. *Clinics in Sports Medicine* 11:351-362.

———. 1998. Too slim, amenorrheic, fracture-prone: The female athlete triad. *ACSM's Health and Fitness Journal* 2:20-25.

Otis, C.L., B. Drinkwater, M. Johnson, A. Louks, and J.H. Wilmore. 1997. American College of Sports Medicine position stand. The female athlete triad: Disordered eating, amenorrhea, and osteoporosis. *Medicine and Science in Sports and Exercise* 29:i-ix.

Otis, C.L., and R. Goldingay. 2000. *The athletic woman's survival guide: How to win the battle against eating disorders, amenorrhea, and osteoporosis.* Champaign, IL: Human Kinetics.

Parente, A.B. 1989. Music as a therapeutic tool in treating anorexia nervosa. In *Experiential therapies for eating disorders*, ed. L.M. Hornyak and E.K. Baker. New York: Guilford.

Parr, R.B., M.A. Porter, and S.C. Hodgson. 1984. Nutrient knowledge and practice of coaches, trainers, and athletes. *Physician and Sportsmedicine* 3:127-138.

Parry-Jones, W.L. 1985. Archival exploration of anorexia nervosa. *Journal of Psychiatric Research* 19 (2/3): 95-100.

Pasman, L., and J.K. Thompson. 1988. Body image and eating disturbance in obligatory runners, obligatory weightlifters and sedentary individuals. *International Journal of Eating Disorders* 7 (6): 759-769.

Paxton, S.J. 1993. A prevention program for disturbed eating and body dissatisfaction in adolescent girls: A 1-year follow-up. *Health Education Research: Theory and Practice* 8:43-51.

Petrie, T.A. 1993. Disordered eating in female collegiate gymnasts: Prevalence and personality/attitudinal correlates. *Journal of Sport and Exercise Psychology* 15:424-436.

———. 1996. Differences between male and female college lean sport athletes, nonlean sport athletes, and non-athletes on behavioral and psychological indices of eating disorders. *Journal of Applied Sport Psychology* 8:218-230.

Petrie, T.A., and S. Stoever. 1993. The incidence of bulimia nervosa and pathogenic weight control behaviors in female collegiate gymnasts. *Research Quarterly of Exercise and Sport* 64 (2): 238-241.

Polivy, J., and I. Federoff. 1997. Group psychotherapy. In *Handbook of treatment for eating disorders*, ed. D.M. Garner and P.E. Garfinkel. New York: Guilford.

Polivy, J., and C.P. Herman. 1985. Dieting and bingeing: A causal analysis. *American Psychologist* 40:193-201.

Pomeroy, C., and J.E. Mitchell. 1992. Medical issues in the eating disorders. In *Eating, body weight and performance in athletes: Disorders of modern society*, ed. K.D. Brownell, J. Rodin, and J.H. Wilmore, 202-221. Philadelphia: Lea and Febiger.

Pope, H.G., A.J. Gruber, P. Choi, R. Olivardia, and K.A. Phillips. 1997. Muscle dysmorphia: An unrecognized form of body dysmorphic disorder. *Psychosomatics* 38:548-557.

Pope, H.G., and D.L. Katz. 1994. Psychiatric and medical effects of anabolic-androgenic steroid use: A controlled study of 160 athletes. *Archives of General Psychiatry* 51:375-382.

Pope, H.G., D.L. Katz, and J.I. Hudson. 1993. Anorexia nervosa and "reverse anorexia" among 108 male body builders. *Comparative Psychiatry* 34:406-409.

Pope, H.G., Jr., K.A. Phillips, and R. Olivardia. 2000. *The Adonis complex: The secret crisis of male body obsession*. New York: Free Press.

Pugliese, M.T., F. Liftshitz, G. Grad, P. Fort, and M. Marks-Katz. 1983. Fear of obesity: A cause for short stature and delayed puberty. *New England Journal of Medicine* 309: 513-518.

Ravussin, E., B. Burnand, Y. Schutz, and E. Jequire. 1982. Twenty-four hour energy expenditure and resting metabolic rate in obese, moderately obese and control subjects. *American Journal of Clinical Nutrition* 35:566-573.

Rice, J.B., M. Hardenbergh, and L.M. Hornyak. 1989. Disturbed body image in anorexia nervosa: Dance/movement therapy interventions. In *Experiential therapies for eating disorders*, ed. L.M. Hornyak and E.K. Baker. New York: Guilford.

Robinson, P.H., and N.L. Holden. 1986. Bulimia nervosa in the male: A report of nine cases. *Psychological Medicine* 16:795-803.

Rodin, J. 1993. Cultural and psychosocial determinants of weight concerns. *Annals of Internal Medicine* 119:643-645.

Rodin, J., and L. Larsen. 1992. Social factors and the ideal body shape. In *Eating, body weight and performance in athletes: Disorders of modern society*, ed. K.D. Brownell, J. Rodin, and J.H. Wilmore, 146-158. Philadelphia: Lea and Febiger.

Rosen, L.W., and D.O. Hough. 1988. Pathogenic weight control behaviors of female college gymnasts. *Physician and Sportsmedicine* 16 (9): 141-144.

Rosen, L.W., D.B. McKeag, D.O. Hough, and V. Curley. 1986. Pathogenic weight control behavior in female athletes. *Physician and Sportsmedicine* 14 (1): 79-95.

Rosenbaum, M., J. Hirsch, E. Murphy, and R.L. Leibel. 2000. Effects of changes in body weight on carbohydrate metabolism, catecholamine excretion, and thyroid function. *American Journal of Clinical Nutrition* 71:1421-1432.

Rosenblum, J., and S. Forman. 2002. Evidence-based treatment of eating disorders. *Current Opinion in Pediatrics* 14:379-383.

Rucinski, A. 1989. Relationship of body image and dietary intake of competitive ice skaters. *Journal of the American Dietetic Association* 89:98-100.

Russell, G. 1979. Bulimia nervosa: An ominous variant of anorexia nervosa. *Psychological Medicine* 9 (3): 429-448.

Ryan, R. 1992a. Management of eating problems in the athletic setting. In *Eating, body weight and performance in athletes: Disorders of modern society*, ed. K. Brownell, J. Rodin, and J.H. Wilmore, 344-362. Philadelphia: Lea and Febiger.

———. 1992b. *The performance team protocol manual*. Austin: University of Texas at Austin, Athletics for Women.

Sacks, M.H. 1990. Psychiatry and sports. *Annals of Sports Medicine* 5:47-52.

Sample, S. 2000. Using weight to control the uncontrollable. *Health Sciences Report, University of Utah* 24 (2): 23-27.

Schmalz, K. 1993. Nutritional beliefs and practices of adolescent athletes. *Journal of School Nursing* 9:18-22.

Schneider, J.A., and W.S. Agras. 1987. Bulimia in males: A matched comparison with females. *International Journal of Eating Disorders* 6:235-242.

Schneider, M., M. Fisher, S. Weinerman, and M. Lesser. 2002. Correlates of low bone density in females with anorexia nervosa. *International Journal of Adolescent Medicine and Health* 14:297-306.

Schulz, L.O., S. Alger, I. Harper, J.H. Wilmore, and E. Ravussin. 1992. Energy expenditure of elite female runners measured by respiratory chamber and doubly-labeled water. *Journal of Applied Physiology* 72:23-28.

Schwenk, T.L. 1997. Psychoactive drugs and athletic performance. *Physician and Sports-medicine* 25 (1): 32-46.

Selby, R., H.M. Weinstein, and T.S. Bird. 1990. The health of university athletes: Attitudes, behaviors, and stressors. *Journal of the American College of Health* 39:11-18.

Shangold, M.M., R. Freeman, B. Thysen, and M. Gatz. 1979. The relationship between long-distance running, plasma progesterone, and luteal phase length. *Fertility and Sterility* 31:130-133.

Shisslak, C.M., M. Crago, and L.S. Estes. 1995. The spectrum of eating disturbances. *International Journal of Eating Disorders* 18:209-219.

Simonsen, J.C., W.M. Sherman, D.R. Lamb, A.R. Dernbach, A.J. Doyle, and R. Strauss. 1991. Dietary carbohydrate, muscle glycogen and power output during rowing training. *Journal of Applied Physiology* 70:1500-1505.

Skinner, R., and A.M. Grooms. 2002. Body composition measurement: A tool for use, not abuse. *SCAN's PULSE* 21:9-11.

Slear, T. 2001. I'm better than this. *Splash* 9:16-19.

Smith, N.J. 1980. Excessive weight loss and food aversion in athletes simulating anorexia nervosa. *Pediatrics* 66:139-142.

Smith-Rockwell, M., S.M. Nickols-Richardson, and F.W. Thye. 2001. Nutrition knowledge, opinions and practices of coaches and athletic trainers at a Division I university. *International Journal of Sport Nutrition and Exercise Metabolism* 11:174-185.

Smolak, L., M.P. Levine, and R. Streigel-Moore, eds. 1996. *The developmental psychopathology of eating disorders: Implications for research, prevention, and treatment.* Manwah, NJ: Lawrence Erlbaum.

Smolak, L., S.K. Murnen, and A.E. Ruble. 2000. Female athletes and eating problems: A meta-analysis. *International Journal of Eating Disorders* 27:371-380.

Soyka, L.A., S. Grinspoon, L.L. Levitsky, D.B. Herzog, and A. Klibanski. 1999. The effects of anorexia nervosa on bone metabolism in female adolescents. *Journal of Clinical Endocrinology and Metabolism* 84:4489-4496.

Stark, A., S. Aronow, and T. McGeehan. 1989. Dance/movement therapy with bulimic patients. In *Experiential therapies for eating disorders*, ed. L.M. Hornyak and E.K. Baker. New York: Guilford.

Steen, S.N., and K.D. Brownell. 1990. Patterns of weight loss and regain in wrestlers: Has the tradition changed? *Medicine and Science in Sports and Exercise* 22:762-768.

Stein, R.L., B.E. Saelens, J.Z. Dounchis, C.M. Lewczyk, A.K. Swenson, and D.E. Wilfley. 2001. Treatment of eating disorders in women. *Counseling Psychologist* 29 (5): 695-732.

Stoutjesdyk, D., and R. Jevne. 1993. Eating disorders among high performance athletes. *Journal of Youth and Adolescence* 22:271-282.

Strauss, R.H., R.R. Lanese, and W.B. Malarkey. 1985. Weight loss in amateur wrestlers and its effects on serum testosterone levels. *Journal of the American Medical Association* 254:3337-3338.

Stunkard, A.J. 1981. "Restrained eating": What it is and a new scale to measure it. In *The body weight regulatory system: Normal and disturbed mechanisms,* ed. L.A. Cioffi et al., 243-251. New York: Raven Press.

Sundgot-Borgen, J. 1993a. Nutrient intakes of elite female athletes suffering from eating disorders. *International Journal of Sport Nutrition* 3:431-442.

———. 1993b. Prevalence of eating disorders in elite female athletes. *International Journal of Sport Nutrition* 3:29-40.

———. 1994. Risk and trigger factors for the development of eating disorders in female athletes. *Medicine and Science in Sports and Exercise* 26:414-419.

———. 1996. Eating disorders, energy intake, training volume, and menstrual function in high-level modern rhythmic gymnasts. *International Journal of Sport Nutrition* 6: 100-109.

———. 1998. Eating disorders. In *Nutrition for exercise and sport,* ed. J.R. Berning and S.N. Steen, 187-204. Gaithersburg, MD: Aspen.

———. 1999. Eating disorders among male and female athletes. *British Journal of Sports Medicine* 33:434.

Sundgot-Borgen, J., and C.B. Corbin. 1987. Eating disorders among female athletes. *Physician and Sportsmedicine* 15 (2): 89-95.

Sundgot-Borgen, J., M. Dlungland, G. Torstveit, and C. Rolland. 1999. Prevalence of eating disorders in male and female elite athletes. *Medicine and Science in Sports and Exercise* 31:S297.

Sundgot-Borgen, J., J.H. Rosenvinge, R. Bahr, and L.S. Schneider. 2002. The effect of exercise, cognitive therapy, and nutritional counseling in treating bulimia. *Medicine and Science in Sports and Exercise* 34 (2): 190-195.

Sykora, C., C.M. Grilo, D.E. Wilfley, and K.D. Brownell. 1993. Eating, weight, and dieting disturbances in male and female lightweight and heavyweight rowers. *International Journal of Eating Disorders* 14:203-211.

Szmukler, G.I. 1983. Weight and food preoccupation in a population of English schoolgirls. In *Understanding anorexia and bulimia,* ed. J.G. Bangman, 21-28. Columbus, OH: Ross Laboratories.

Szmukler, G.I., I. Eisler, C. Gillies, and M.E. Hayward. 1985. The implications of anorexia nervosa in a ballet school. *Journal of Psychiatric Research* 19:177-181.

Tanner, S.M. 1994. Preparticipation examination targeted for the female athlete. *Clinics in Sports Medicine* 13 (2): 330-353.

Taub, D.E., and E.M. Blinde. 1992. Eating disorders among adolescent female athletes: Influence of athletic participation and sport team membership. *Adolescence* 27:833-848.

Terry, P.C., A.M. Lane, and L. Warren. 1999. Eating attitudes, body shape perceptions, and mood of elite rowers. *Journal of Science and Medicine in Sport* 2:67-72.

Thelen, M.H., J. Farmer, S. Wonderlich, and M. Smith. 1991. A revision of the bulimia test: The BULIT-R. *Journal of Consulting and Clinical Psychology* 3:119-124.

Thien, V., A. Thomas, D. Markin, and C.L. Birmingham. 2000. Pilot study of a graded exercise program for the treatment of anorexia nervosa. *International Journal of Eating Disorders* 28:101-106.

Thompson, J.L., and M.M. Manore. 1996. Effects of diet and diet-plus-exercise programs on resting metabolic rate: A meta-analysis. *International Journal of Sport Nutrition* 6:41-61.

Thompson, J., M.M. Manore, and J.S. Skinner. 1993. Resting metabolic rate and thermic effect of a meal in low- and adequate-energy intake male endurance athletes. *International Journal of Sport Nutrition* 3:194-206.

Thompson, K.J., and P. Blanton. 1987. Energy conservation and exercise dependence: A sympathetic arousal hypothesis. *Medicine and Science in Sports and Exercise* 19: 91-99.

Thompson, R.A., and R.T. Sherman. 1993. *Helping athletes with eating disorders.* Champaign, IL: Human Kinetics.

Tiggemann, J., and A.S. Pickering. 1996. Role of television in adolescent women's body dissatisfaction and drive for thinness. *International Journal of Eating Disorders* 20: 199-203.

Tuschl, R.J., P. Platte, R.G. Laessle, W. Stichler, and K.M. Pirke. 1990. Energy expenditure and everyday eating behavior in healthy young women. *American Journal of Clinical Nutrition* 52:81-86.

Walberg, J.L., and C.S. Johnston. 1991. Menstrual function and eating behavior in female recreational weight lifters and competitive body builders. *Medicine and Science in Sports and Exercise* 23:30-36.

Waller, M., and E. Haymes. 1996. The effects of heat and exercise on sweat iron losses. *Medicine and Science in Sports and Exercise* 28:197-203.

Ward, A., N. Brown, and J. Treasure. 1997. Persistent osteopenia after recovery from anorexia nervosa. *International Journal of Eating Disorders* 22:71-75.

Warren, M.P., and S. Shanmugan. 2000. The female athlete. *Bailliere's Clinical Endocrinology and Metabolism* 14:37-53.

Weaver, C.M., and S. Rajaram. 1992. Exercise and iron status. *Journal of Nutrition* 122: 782-787.

Webb, S.M., and M. Puig-Domingo. 1995. Role of melatonin in health and disease. *Clinical Endocrinology* 42:221-234.

Weight, L.M., and T.D. Noakes. 1987. Is running an analogue to anorexia? A survey of the incidence of eating disorders in female distance runners. *Medicine and Science in Sports and Exercise* 19:213-216.

Weinsier, R., G. Hunter, and Y. Schutz. 2001. Metabolic response to weight loss. *American Journal of Clinical Nutrition* 73:655.

Weissinger, E., T.J. Housh, G.O. Johnson, and S.A. Evans. 1991. Weight loss behavior in high school wrestling: Wrestler and parent perceptions. *Pediatric Exercise Science* 3:64-73.

Weyer, C., R.L. Walford, I.T. Harper, M. Milner, T. MacCallum, P.A. Tataranni, and E. Ravussin. 2000. Energy metabolism after 2 y of energy restriction: The Biosphere 2 experiment. *American Journal of Clinical Nutrition* 72:946-953.

Wilkens, J.A., F.J. Boland, and J. Albinson. 1991. A comparison of male and female university athletes and non-athletes on eating disorder indices: Are athletes protected? *Journal of Sport Behavior* 14:129-143.

Williams, M.H. 2001. *Nutrition for fitness and sport.* 6th ed. Boston: McGraw Hill.

Williams, N.I., J.C. Young, J.W. McArther, B. Bullen, G.S. Skinar, and B. Turnbull. 1995. Strenuous exercise with caloric restriction: Effect on leutinizing hormone secretion. *Medicine and Science in Sports and Exercise* 27:1390-1398.

Williamson, D.A. 1990. *Assessment of eating disorders: Obesity, anorexia and bulimia nervosa.* New York: Pergamon Press.

Williamson, D.A., R.G. Netemeyer, L.P. Jackman, D.A. Anderson, C.L. Funsch, and J.Y. Rabalais. 1995. Structural equation modeling for risks for the development of eating disorder symptoms in female athletes. *International Journal of Eating Disorders* 4: 387-393.

Wilmore, J.H. 1991. Eating and weight disorders in the female athlete. *International Journal of Sport Nutrition* 1:104-107.

———. 1992. Body weight standards and athletic performance. In *Eating, body weight and performance in athletes: Disorders of modern society,* ed. K.D. Brownell, J. Rodin, and J.H. Wilmore, 315-329. Philadelphia: Lea and Febiger.

Wilmore, J.H., K.C. Wambsgans, M. Brenner, C.E. Broeder, I. Paijmans, J.A. Volpe, and K.A. Wilmore. 1992. Is there energy conservation in amenorrheic compared with eumenorrheic distance runners? *Journal of Applied Physiology* 72:15-22.

Wilson, G.T., and W.S. Agras. 2001. Practice guidelines for eating disorders. *Behavior Therapy* 32:219-234.

Wiseman, C.V., J.J. Gray, J.E. Mosimann, and A.H. Ahrens. 1992. Cultural expectations of thinness in women: An update. *International Journal of Eating Disorders* 11:85-89.

Wolman, R.L., P. Clark, E. McNally, M. Harries, and J. Reeve. 1990. Menstrual state and exercise as determinants of spinal and trabecular bone density in female athletes. *British Medical Journal* 301:516-518.

Woodside, D., D. Garner, W. Rockert, and P. Garfinkel. 1990. Insights from a clinical and psychometric comparison with female patients. In *Males with eating disorders,* ed. A. Andersen, 100-115. New York: Brunner/Mazel.

www.ltspeed.com/bjblindr/anmeddis.htm. 2003. Anorexia nervosa in association with medical disorders. 21 June.

Zeigler, P., S. Nensley, J.B. Roepke, S.H. Whitaker, B.W. Craig, and A. Drewnowski. 1998. Eating attitudes and energy intakes of female skaters. *Medicine and Science in Sports and Exercise* 30:583-586.

Zetin, M., and D. Tate. 1999. *The psychopharmacology sourcebook.* Los Angeles: Lowell House.

index

Note: The italicized *f* and *t* following page numbers refer to figures and tables, respectively.

about the author

Katherine Beals, PhD, RD, is currently employed by Fleishman-Hillard International Communications, where she directs the scientific affairs for clients in the food and agribusiness division.

Prior to joining Fleishman-Hillard, Dr. Beals held the rank of associate professor of nutrition at Ball State University in Muncie, Indiana. During her seven-year tenure at Ball State, Dr. Beals taught courses in macro- and micronutrient metabolism; sport nutrition; and energy balance, obesity, and weight control. She also served as the nutritional consultant to the intercollegiate athletic program.

Dr. Beals has been providing nutritional counseling to athletes and active individuals with eating disorders for more than 10 years. Dr. Beals has authored numerous articles on disordered eating in athletes and frequently presents on the subject. A competitive athlete for more than 20 years in distance running, swimming, and triathlons, Dr. Beals has seen disordered eating firsthand in both teammates and competitors.

Dr. Beals is a Fellow of the American College of Sports Medicine (ACSM) and a member of the Academy of Eating Disorders (AED), the American Dietetic Association (ADA), and both the Research and Sports, Cardiovascular, Wellness, and Eating Disorders (SCAN) practice groups of ADA. She also serves as editor of the newsletter for the Research practice group of ADA, nutrition editor of *ACSMs Fit Society* newsletter and sports nutrition editor for SCANs newsletter the *PULSE*.

Dr. Beals earned her PhD in exercise science and physical education from Arizona State University. She is also a registered dietitian.